Lois and Bill,

11-7-13

In Divine Light
and Love!
Love you so Much!

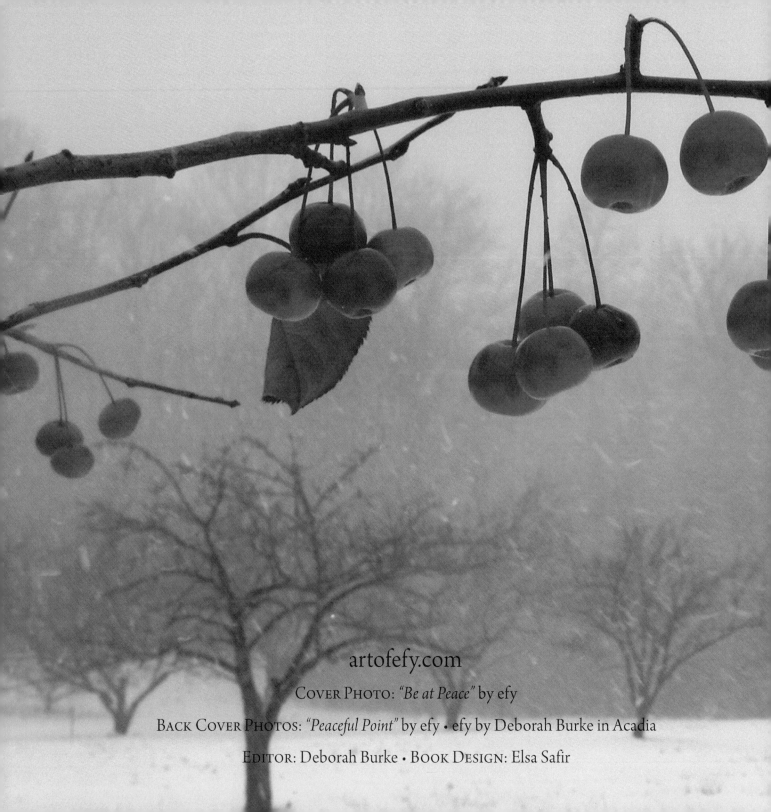

artofefy.com

Cover Photo: *"Be at Peace"* by efy

Back Cover Photos: *"Peaceful Point"* by efy • efy by Deborah Burke in Acadia

Editor: Deborah Burke • Book Design: Elsa Safir

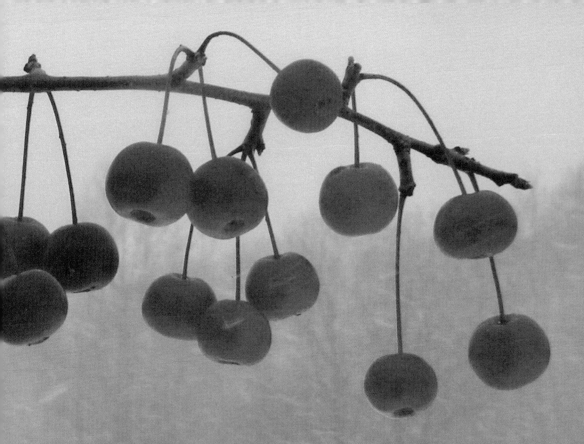

Healing Through Divine Light

A Journey In Photos by efy

Tidings

For my son, who had to sacrifice so much so I could heal
and become whole. May you understand how much
love it took for me to change our lives forever.
I love you!

Contents

Prelude

I was in a very thin time – at my weakest and most desperate – when the journey told through these photographs and journal writings began. But the story begins even earlier. As a child, I loved to color. My inner nudging guided me to paint on a kind of make-shift artist's easel. No one ever really noticed or told me to keep it up, but I loved the experience of placing colors on paper.

And I loved spending hours outdoors, climbing those huge old trees in our yard as far up as I could go. I'd sit up there at the top and take in everything. I especially loved the birds. I'd lose track of time. I was never ready to go in, until forced by darkness.

In elementary school, I began taking photos of our family dogs with a small Kodak camera. My dog, Togo, was a beautiful white Husky. In the early 1980s, a friend introduced me to the amazing 35mm camera. I had to have my own. That is when my life as a nature photographer began.

I felt at home in nature – at the top of a tree, under bending branches, in the middle of the woods, or standing near a flowing stream. Each moment a new frame: water flowing over shale or red and yellow maple leaves falling quietly into a creek.

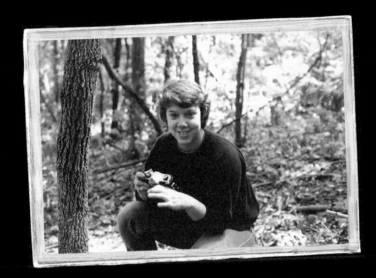

Here I am with my new 35mm camera in one of my favorite spots, the woods near my hometown. In the 1980s, I was known as Lynda, my given name.

In 1997, I began to experience symptoms that became increasingly troublesome. I tripped all the time. I couldn't find my way home from the grocery store. Once, I didn't recognize my husband when he walked out of our garage. When I fell into bed at night, pains shot through my body and head. I prayed that I would never wake up.

It wasn't until mid-May 2003, that I was diagnosed with severe Lyme disease. It robbed me of my body as I had known it, took all my athletic ability from me, and devastated my mind.

Lyme disease forced me to put away my camera. It hurt too much to lift it. I felt like an invalid, exhausted all the time and trapped. Even my ears hurt. As the shooting pains intensified, I felt as though I was dying. I was afraid for myself, for my husband, and for my young son.

Author Note: The text in *italics* represents my journal writings.

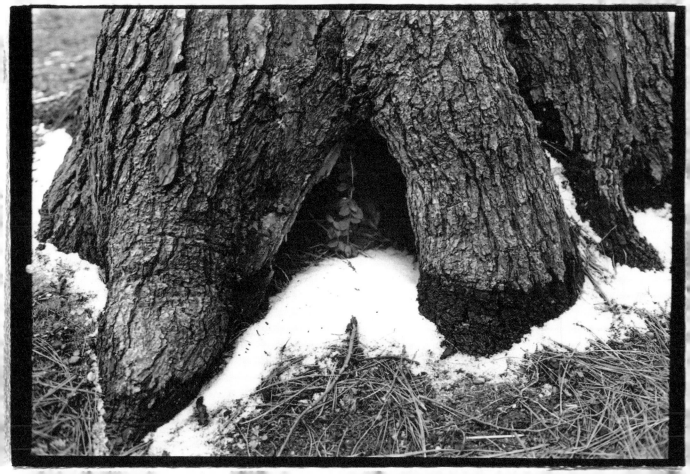

Reiki gathering out of desperation – though I had no idea what Reiki was.

The Reiki treatment took place at HeartSong, a spiritual retreat center deep in the woods in central Ohio. The main floor was nearly level with the tops of the trees in the woods that surrounded it. At one end, a warm fire crackled in the big stone fireplace. It was there that my friends and I gathered to share a meal.

When Jenny, the Reiki master, hurried in from a previous engagement, it seemed as though she was almost blown in the door. She introduced herself and seemed warm, caring, and kind as she explained how Reiki works as a healing modality.

Jenny was serious and spoke softly. She had a quiet intelligence and a deep knowledge as she spoke about individuals who carry hurts from childhood and the pain left by the trauma of abuse. I sat there remembering my childhood. I felt guilt and shame. All I wanted was to feel better.

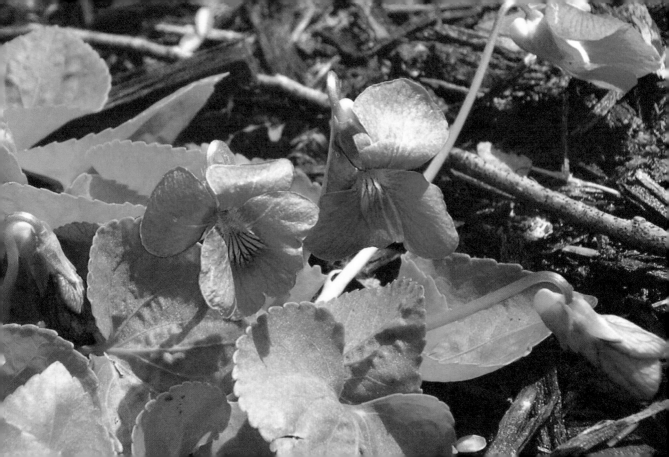

Calming music played as I lay on a table for my first Reiki treatment. I learned that Reiki is the energy of the universe. I lay on my back, my head on a pillow, fully clothed, a light blanket over me. Jenny laid her hands gently on my head first and then went down my whole body to my feet. It was relaxing and when it ended about thirty minutes later, I knew I wanted more.

Although my friends didn't know it, my desperate decision to attend this gathering was triggered by an inner, urgent, last-ditch effort to save my own life. Who would have guessed that one choice and one more try on one ordinary day would change my life forever and my family's as well. My husband, son, and friends would all be changed by what happened. But the biggest change would be within me.

The medical bills from my illness had piled up. I had been on antibiotics for three years. For ten weeks, I had been on heavy doses through an I-V. I spoke with my husband about Reiki and my feeling that it held something for me that regular medical treatment did not. He agreed that I should try it. I talked to Jenny and she was willing to see me for Reiki twice a week and accept what I could pay. I had absolutely no idea that I was beginning to embark on a journey that would forever change my life.

Jenny and I set a time for my first Reiki appointment. I was nervous. Jenny and I both lived on the edge of town, not far from one another. As I drove over the winding hills to her home and then up her long driveway, my heart pounded.

I got to the door and could see Jenny, through the glass, sitting in a rocking chair, with a blanket around her shoulders. *Do I just go in, do I knock?*

Standing there, I questioned my decision to choose Reiki. What was I thinking? I noticed a black Lab curled up on a futon in the middle of the room. I had two black Labs at home and loved them. I relaxed. I knew anyone with a black Lab must be okay.

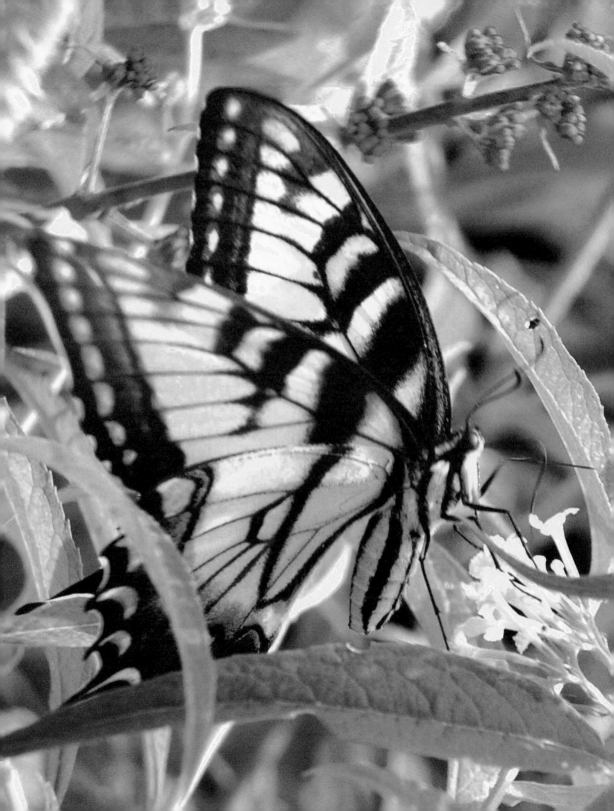

I took this photo of a butterfly during one of the worst days of my illness. Becoming one with the butterfly bush, standing, watching, waiting, among the butterflies and bees on a very hot day, enabled me to capture this image. That day, I needed to be outside, in nature. I was trying to grasp some essence of my former, healthy self. I got the shot and called it "Peace Butterfly."

Peace Butterfly

I gifted Jenny with "Peace Butterfly" at that first appointment. She appreciated it and introduced me to her black Lab, Carly. This is how it began.

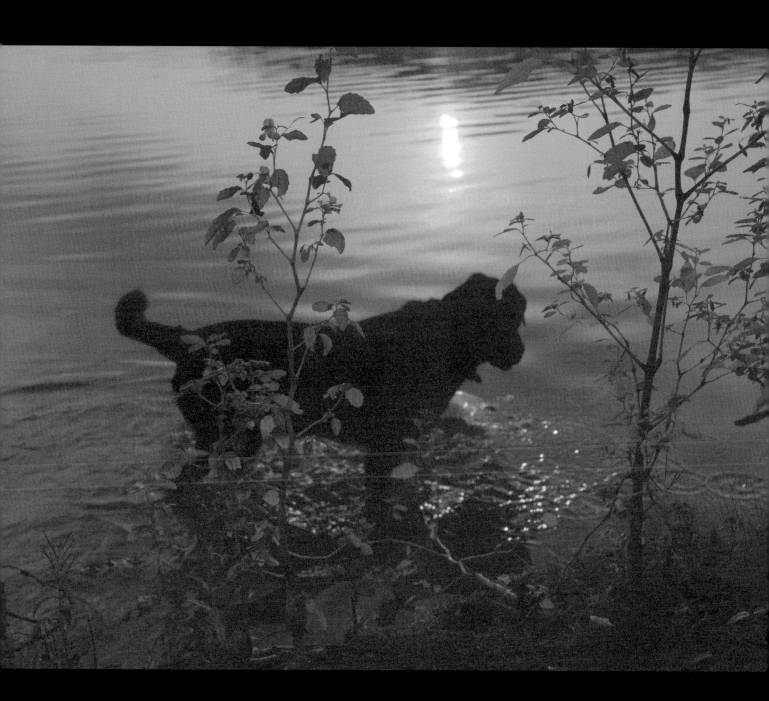

Namaste

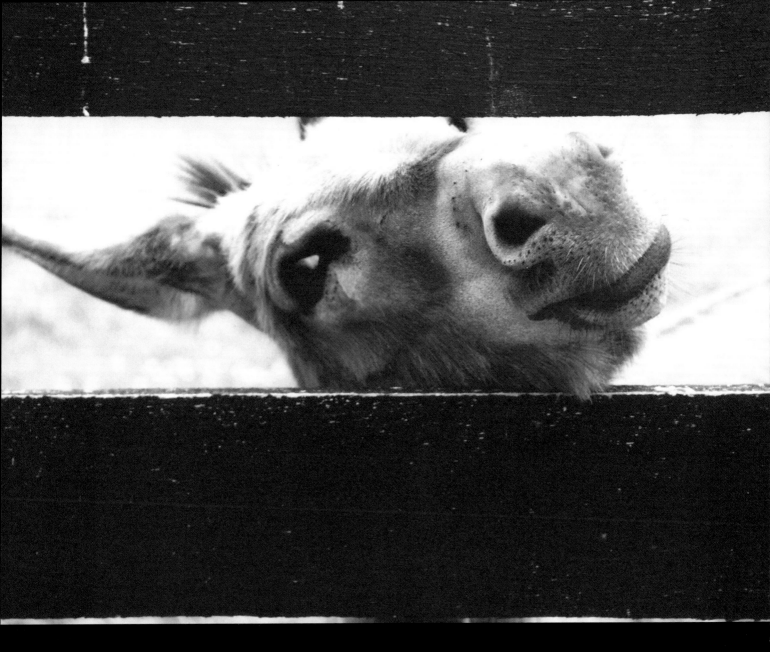

Bongo

My little donkey, Bongo, was a quirky guy. He was a miniature donkey and just the right size for our son at the time. The horses were so big and scary for a little boy. Bongo and two horses made up our little mini-farm on four acres of land. And, depending on the season, we might have a pig or steer for our son's 4H projects. I loved to nuzzle Bongo's soft nose. I could watch him for hours. When the horses lay down in the field to sleep, Bongo would take a stick and poke them until they woke up and played with him.

On my second visit for Reiki, Jenny told me about a natural Spring on a lake near HeartSong. She called it a "healing" Spring. I choose to capitalize the Spring because it has played such an important role in my healing. It almost feels to me like a kindred spirit.

"Would you like to go?" Jenny asked.

"How far? How do we get there?" I was afraid of the shooting pains that would cripple my body. I was afraid of the deer ticks in the woods that had been the source of the Lyme disease.

"By water or a nice long hike in the woods," she said.

I decided to try the hike. I had begun to walk around the track at the local high school after I dropped off my son at school in the morning. At first I couldn't do more than one or two slow laps around the track. I would go home exhausted. Two months later, although not completely healed, I was feeling stronger.

Something inside encouraged me – like a new nudging
– to try the hike to the Spring. I had been so sidelined,
so much like an invalid. I wanted to ditch that person I'd
become and get back to the "old" me who was strong and
healthy. I did not want to be denied.

On the last Sunday in October, my husband and son stood
with me, supporting me, as I headed out for the hike to
the Spring. They didn't know – and neither did I – that
this was the beginning of goodbye.

Before leaving the house, I reached for the 35mm camera
that I hadn't been able to use for so long. I was surprised
that I could pick it up without pains shooting through
my arms and hands. Twenty-four hours after my second
Reiki treatment, I had no pain. Although this respite
lasted for only a short while, it felt great to pick up my
camera again.

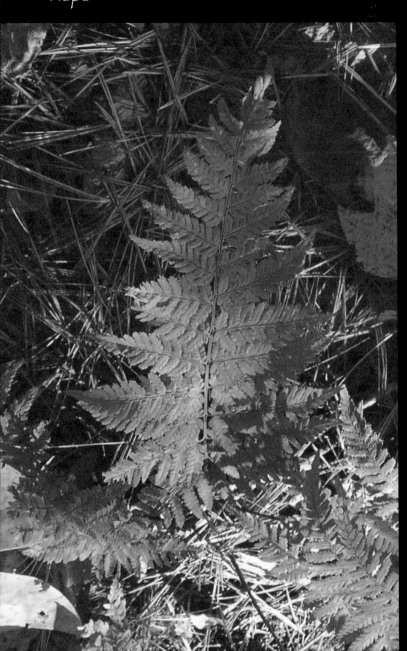

Light was streaming across and through the woods highlighting the beauty as we started the long hike to the Spring. On the way, the shooting pains began and I had to rest. Jenny didn't judge me or grow weary of my need to rest. She seemed not to worry. We went to the Spring that first time on my body's time – and I began to love my body for what it could do.

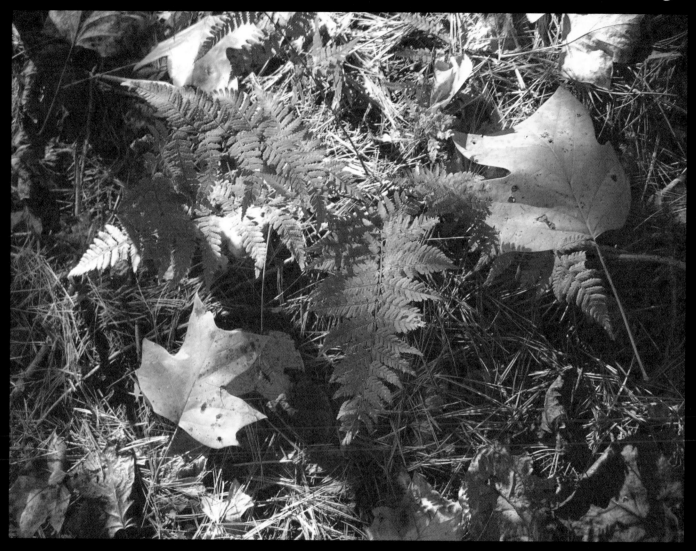

These photos were taken on my first walk to the Spring
when the lighting was streaming across and through the
woods highlighting the beauty of everything in its path.

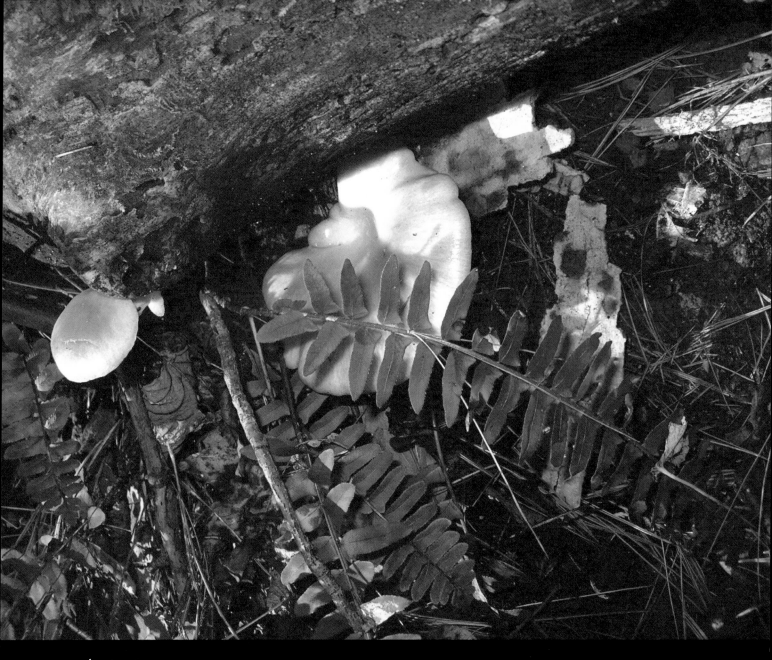

Wonder

I love the contrast of the fern against the fungi in the photo to the left – the way it forms a triangle drew me in. Sometimes it is the simplest elements in nature that call to me to take the photo.

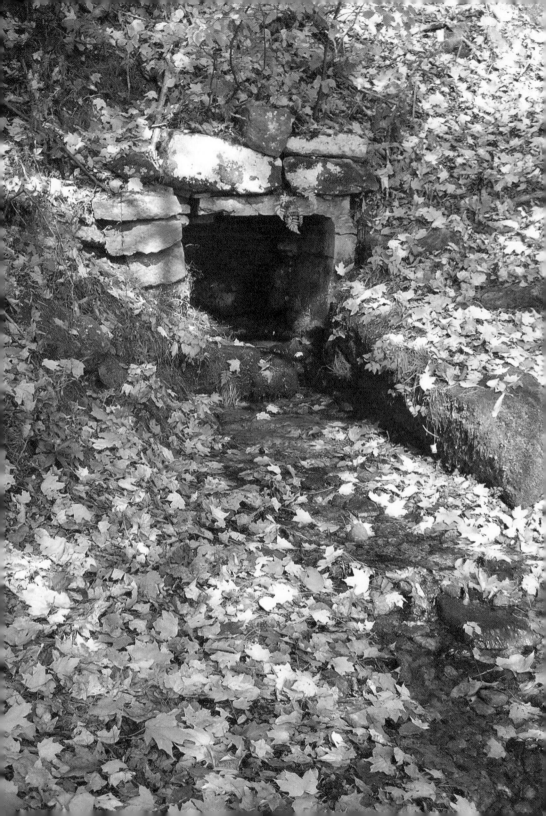

Had only a few Reiki treatments from a
woman I had just met done this? Even
though my legs gave me trouble on the walk
to the Spring, I was able to take photographs.
I began to notice how light fell in the woods.
I was thrilled to be inspired again.

It felt like a new day.

This is the entrance to the Spring. It was
autumn when I first saw it; autumn leaves
sprinkled their carpet of color.
I was smitten.

Jenny explained the protocol observed when approaching a sacred site such as this. She told me to ask permission to approach the Spring and wait for an answer – felt or sensed within me. I could dip my hand in its well and drink from it. I should leave some kind of natural gift at the Spring before departing as a sign of gratitude. I honored this tradition.

In the upper center of this photo is the basin that collects the water that flows from the Spring deep within the hillside. The basin is surrounded by stone. I feel so incredibly blessed to have been to the Spring that October morning – the Spring did herself proud. The light on the beautiful fall leaves was amazing.

Each time I went to the Spring, I would dunk my head in the basin three times and pray for the shooting pains to stop. I took a cupped handful of its water and placed it on my chest. I was trying to be cleansed of the pain that was ravaging my body.

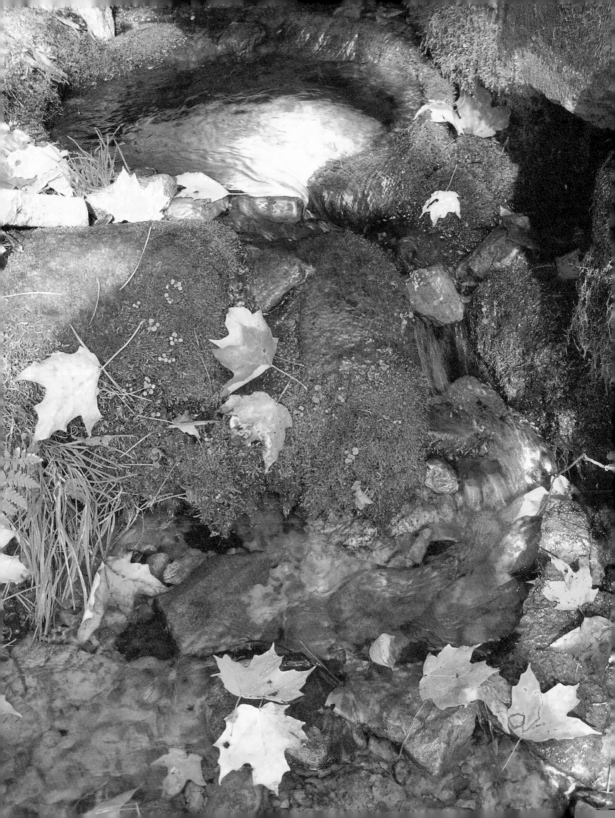

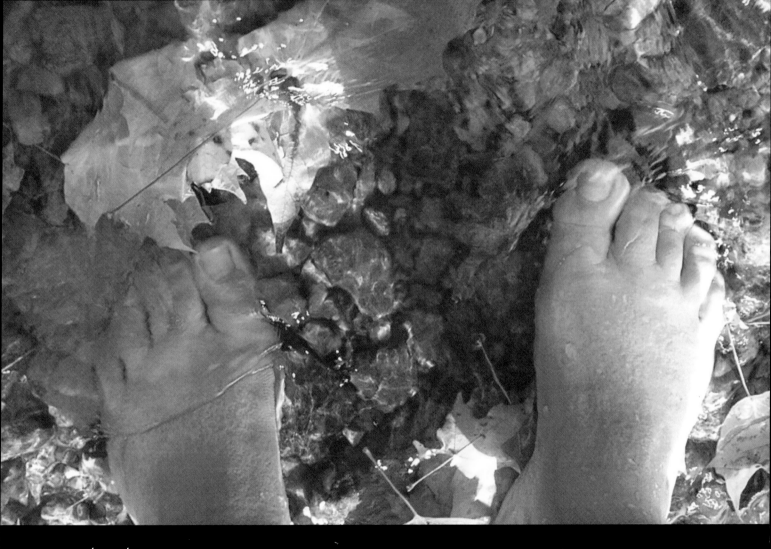

Cherish

What a day this was! I was happy! On my first visit to the Spring, I felt moved to take off my hiking boots and stand in the cold water, and then to capture my feet. The energy took hold of me in ways I've never felt before. As the spring waters flowed out and into the lake, it was so beautiful. I had the best time taking photos at the Spring.

The image of my feet in the cold water on the first of many trips to the Spring is one of my favorite images. It had been so long since I had felt this happy. What was happening to me?

I could have never guessed how important the Spring would become to me. As I took these photos, I had no idea what I was actually capturing with my camera. The Spring is so much more to me than just a place to take photos. It represents healing. It's a sacred place.

When it was time to leave, I faced the Spring. I thanked it and put saliva on four fingers and gently touched the stone to bless it in a prayer of gratitude. Over the years when I've gone to the Spring, I've left strands of hair, a bit of saliva, and many tears, mostly of joy.

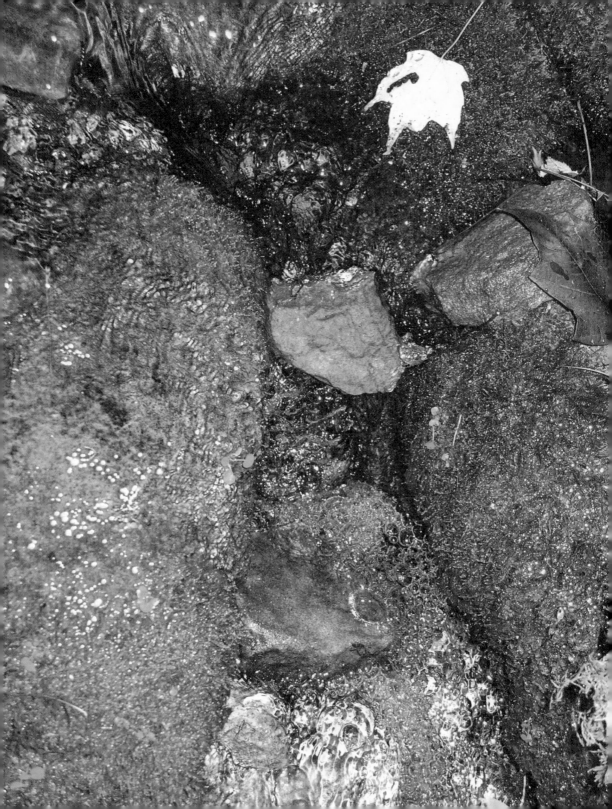

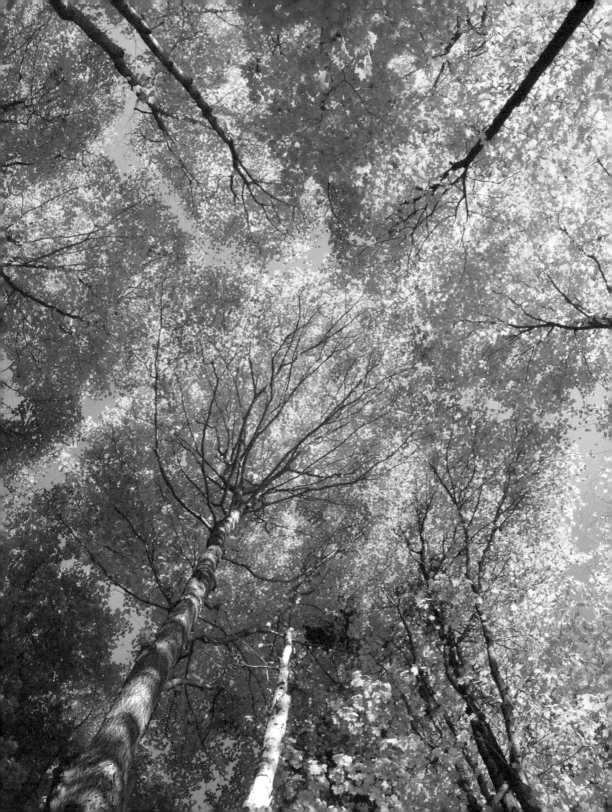

After my first visit to the Spring, I was happy to get home and put the images on my computer and print them. I couldn't wait to share the photos with Jenny on my next Reiki visit. She loved my photos so much that she asked for some of the prints to put up at HeartSong.

Jenny became a good and trusted friend. She became one of my healers. The Spring became one of my healers, and nature too, in amazing ways, healed me. Finally, little by little, bit by bit, in fits and starts, I became my own healer.

A few weeks later, on a trip to the Spring, Jenny invited me to receive Reiki One. She explained that as I learned the basic elements of Reiki, it would be helpful for my healing. I accepted her invitation.

In a ceremony at the Spring, I received the gift of Reiki One, which empowered me to take part in my own healing. I was so taken in by everything new to me that day that I forgot to get out my camera! I never took one photo!

I went to the Spring as often as I could. On the day I took these photos, I felt drawn to the flowing water. It looked and felt like a divine presence, like nature was telling me, *"You are not alone. Everything will be okay!"*

I received Reiki from Jenny twice a week, from October through December. I continued to walk every morning around the track. I gave myself Reiki every day. I began to feel different, better. Around Thanksgiving, I decided to stop taking the antibiotics my doctor had prescribed for Lyme disease.

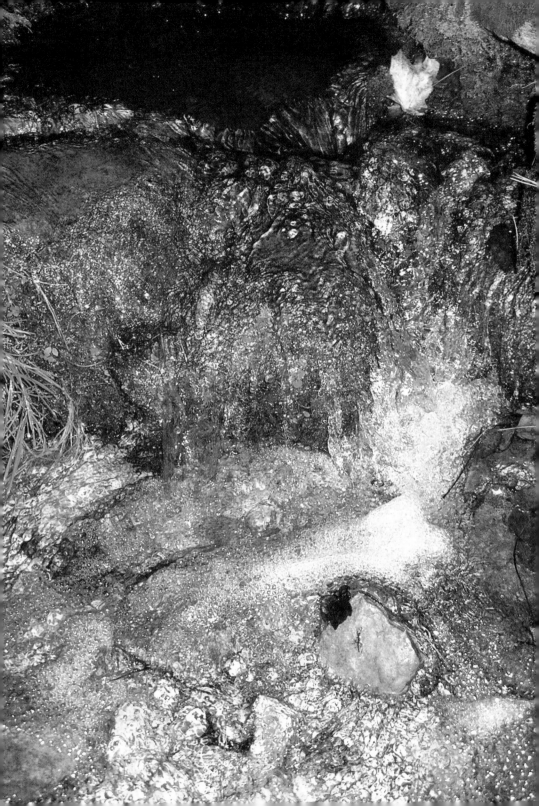

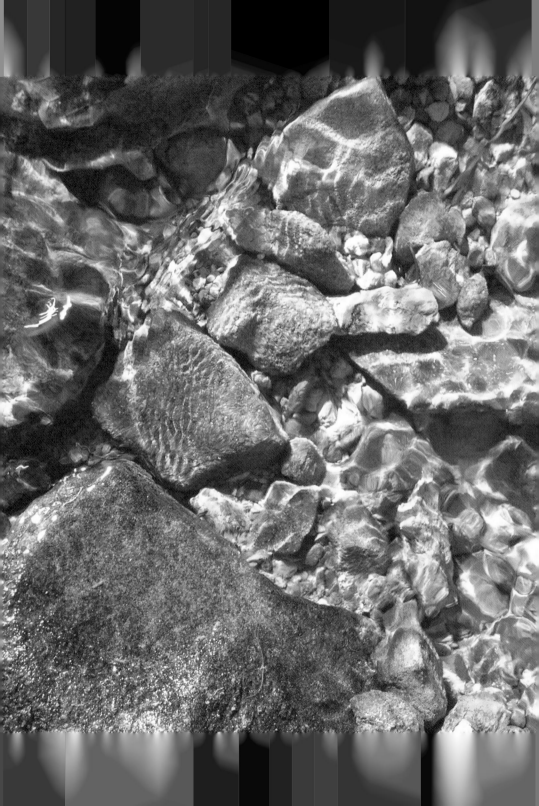

Two months later I went to Pennsylvania for an appointment with my doctor, who specialized in Lyme disease. He was amazed at how much better I was doing. I never told him about the Reiki because I was embarrassed; it wasn't "medical." Nor did I tell him that I had stopped taking the antibiotics. He told me that he had done everything he could for me. "Call if you need to," he said, promising to be there if I needed further treatment.

I've never gone back. I've never needed to go back. I had gotten better. Not healed, just better. This body I could live with. I still had many symptoms, but I was beginning to live again.

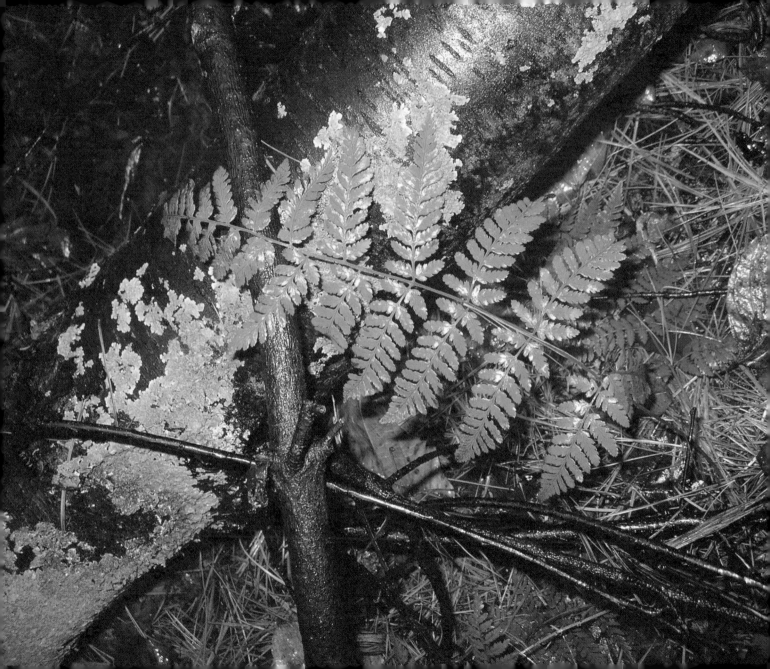

Every time I went to the Spring that fall and winter, I took photographs. I was never without my camera. I now know that I was beginning to beat Lyme disease by becoming present to my body and to my daily life. I received Reiki twice a week for a year.

Not only was I feeling better but I was beginning to change inside also. Something was changing in me – that's all I knew. For awhile.

I had always feared that the God I'd grown up with would ask me to change my life. I never understood where this thought came from. HA! It was true, though. What I came to know as the Divine was asking me to change – and to change in a big way.

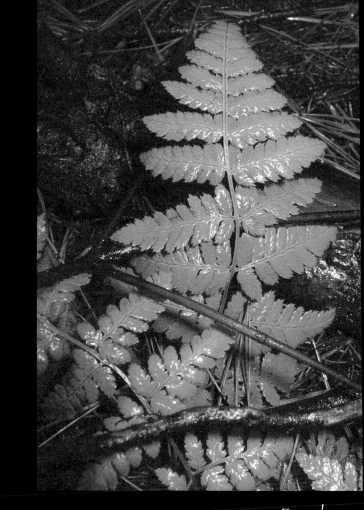

Frond

I know now that I was being called. Here, at the beginning of my healing from Lyme disease, another calling was presenting itself. How it unfolded was so unusual. Or was it?

I'll never forget that morning when I was walking at the high school track and my mind was racing about childhood hurts that were beginning to come up during my Reiki sessions. As I rounded the track, I couldn't believe that I saw angels all along the brick wall by the bleachers. More angels were in the stands! Angels were everywhere. It was as though they were applauding me. Me? I wasn't sure what was happening.

Is this a leaf lodged inside the Spring? Or an angel? From the day I saw the angels around the high school running track, I believe I was being opened up in ways unimaginable. My spirit was coming alive amidst all the turmoil within. I began to trust.

Angel Leaf

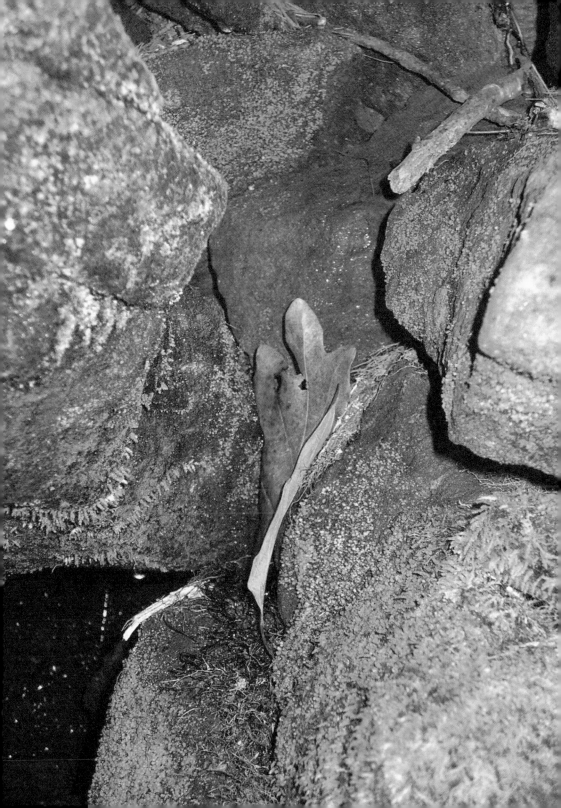

I continued to see the angels. They looked like beings of light, with wings. Most of them were feminine – somehow I knew that. One was masculine and I sensed he was the "guardian." Their voices were so high pitched that while I would sometimes hear them talking, I often couldn't understand what they were saying. One day I heard and understood them: "You have to pay attention to your life, to your calling," they said. "Pay attention to this very moment."

I told Jenny about the angels. She listened with that loving intent. Then she asked if she could walk with me sometime, which felt so supportive. So we would walk and walk and talk with long periods of silence. The image "Gratitude," was taken at the Spring on a chilly day. I shed my shoes and knelt down in the water's flow. The way the water rippled over the stones and leaves and the sunlight washed over all, spoke to my heart. It seemed to be saying, *Give Thanks.*

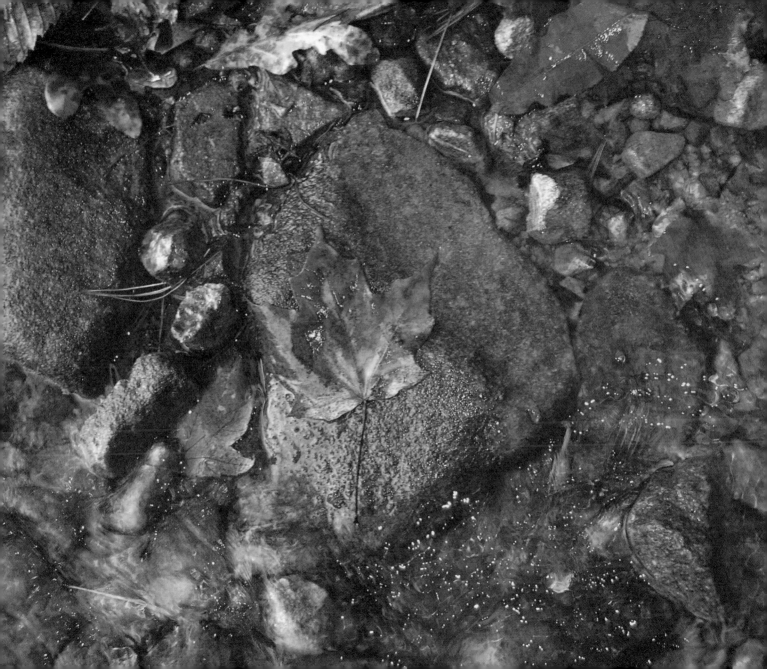

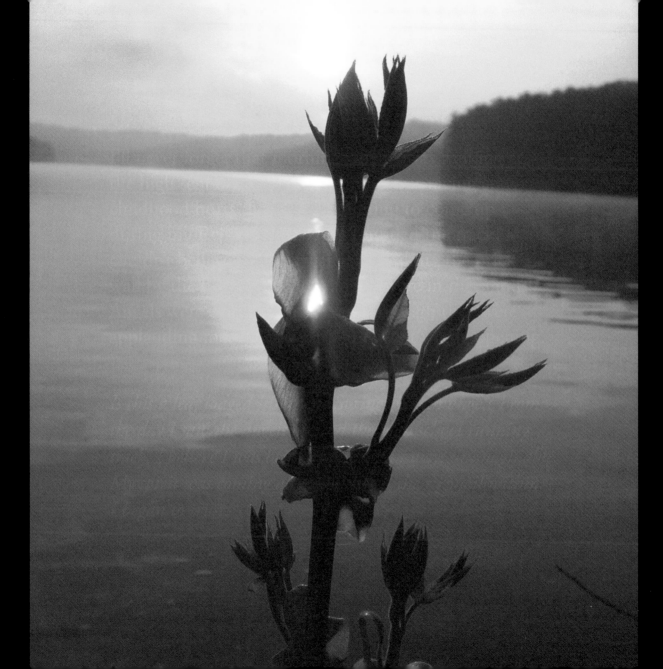

Along with the healing of my body and my inner changes, I noticed that my images were changing too. Before I took a photo, I began to ask permission from the fern, the leaf, the water, the flower.

I'm noticing – and trying to understand – this feeling of the subject "asking" me to take the photo. I wonder if Reiki has opened me to the nature spirits – the energies of the woods in which I was immersing myself. More and more often, there are energies, wisps of light, vague outlines of other beings appearing in my photos that have never been there before. Or is it just that I am noticing them for the first time?

I heard nature asking me to take a photo – not audibly of course – but through my intuition, like a head to heart knowing. I honored nature by asking permission before taking the photo. In return, nature reached out to me, granting beautiful shots. Nature and I connected at a very deep level.

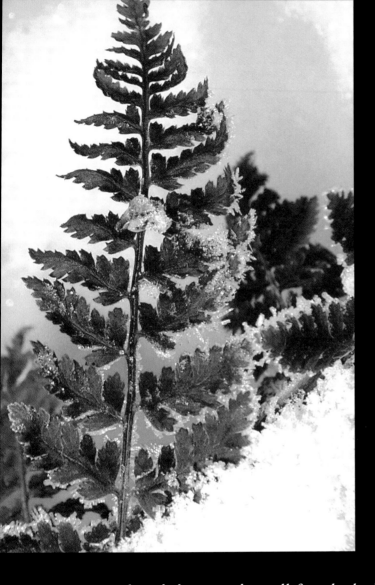

Courage

I was off the antibiotics for Lyme disease, so the only real "healing" in my life at that time was from Reiki and my own work in becoming conscious. I believe the Reiki was opening me up to the universal energies and spirit.

I've never stopped seeing and hearing the nature spirits and the angels. They are everywhere. I trust this gift. It's happened for years now. I no longer need to explain it to myself or try to understand it. It just *is*.

I loved the way this tall fern looked as it was surrounded by snow. It was majestic and beautiful. I was learning what courage meant. This fern in winter seemed to say "Courage!"

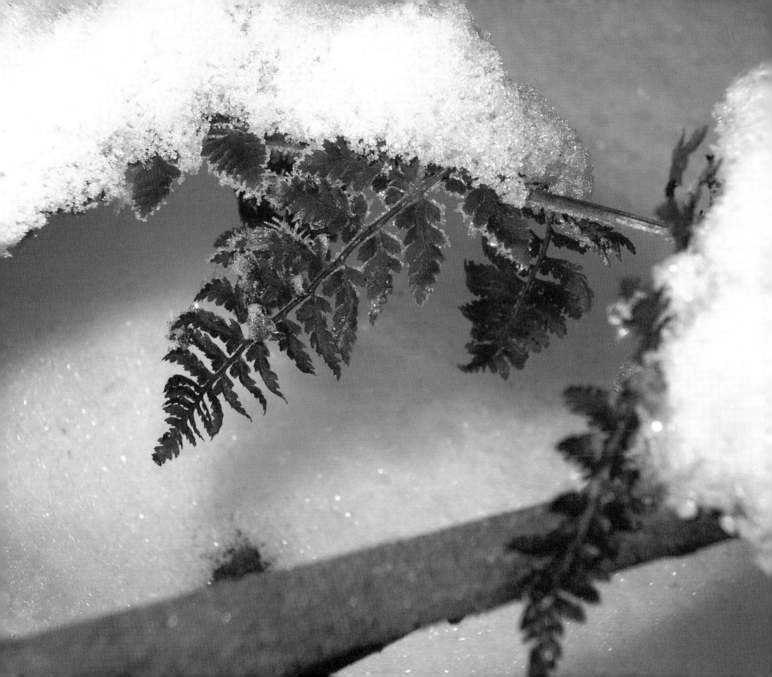

On a retreat at HeartSong that first winter,
I felt more relaxed than I'd ever remember
feeling – ever. This image mirrored
the peacefulness I felt inside. At first, I
thought the wonderful feeling of being so
"at home" was about being at HeartSong.
Later, I realized it was because I was in
nature, among the trees. The trees loved
me – I could feel it. They accepted me,
without judgment.

Solemn Gaze

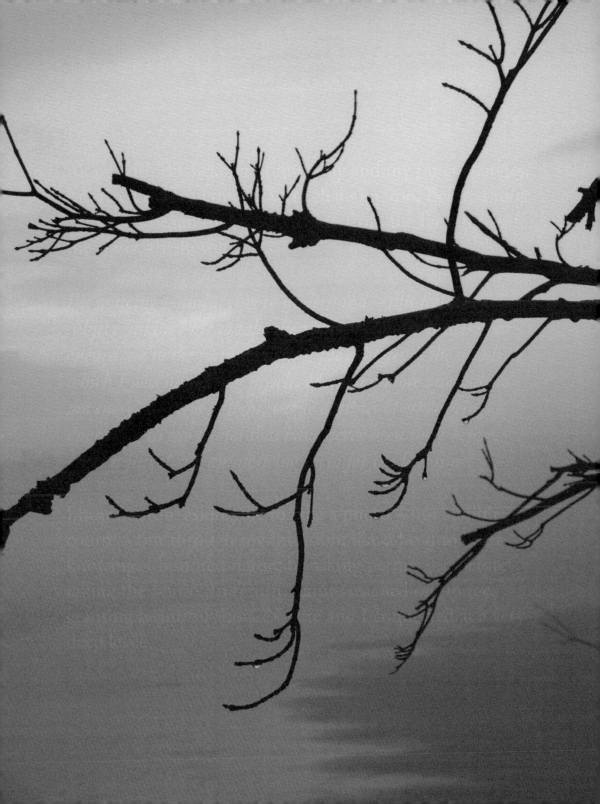

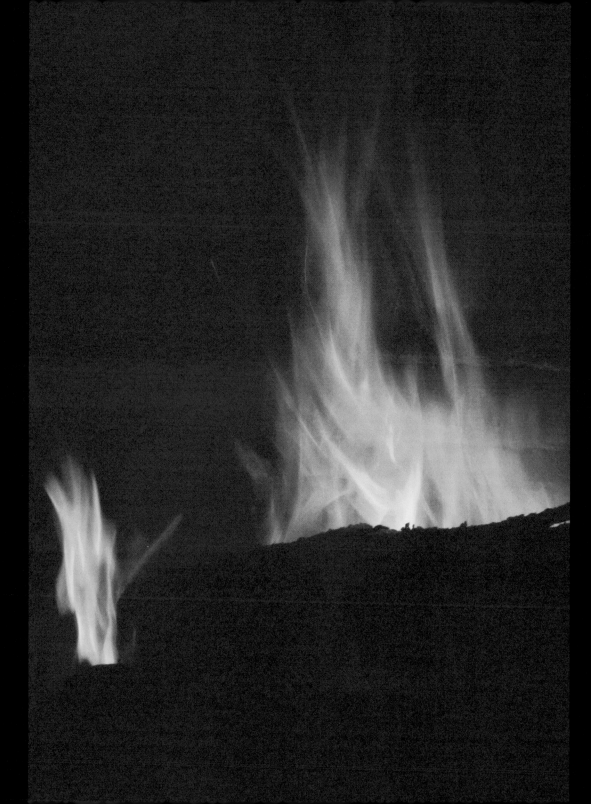

As I stared at the fire in the big stone fireplace at HeartSong, I grabbed my camera. The flames were beautiful as they danced around the logs! But it wasn't until I printed the image that I saw the angels in it. I was stunned when I saw the little fire *"Angel"* conductor out in front conducting the orchestra of flames, arms up in praise.

Fire Angel Conductor

When I couldn't get to the Spring, I missed it. I felt "at home" there. I yearned for that feeling that I had when I went there – the feeling that *It's going to be okay*. I returned to the Spring, time and time again.

Eventually, I moved to the woods by the lake, near the Spring.

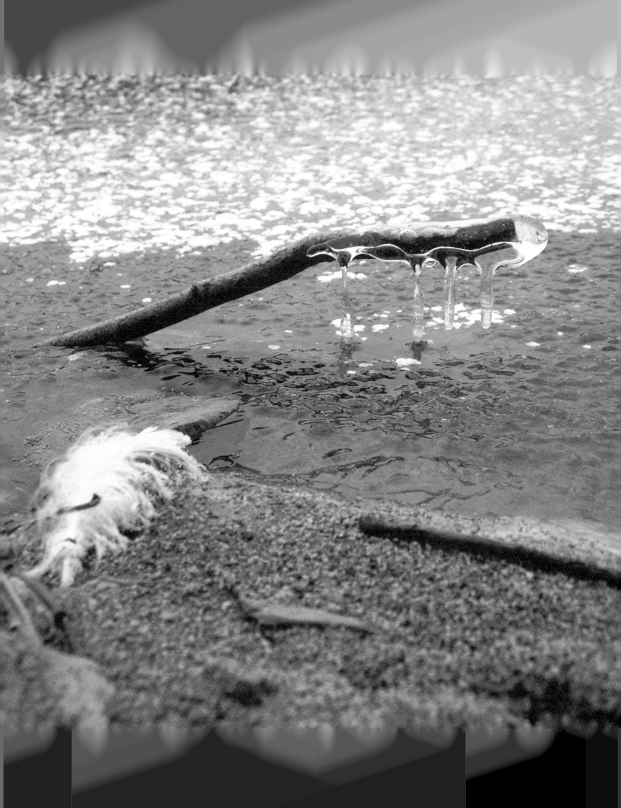

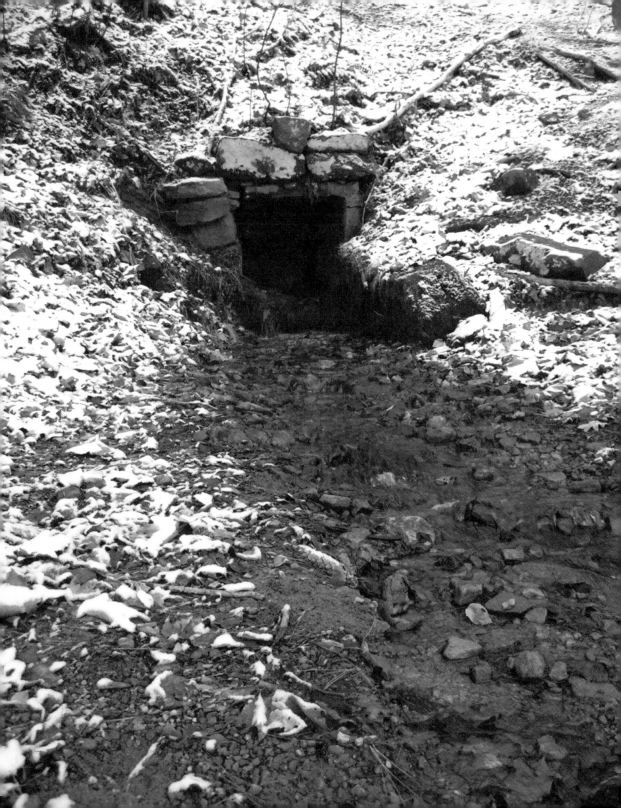

As I hiked around the woods and around the
Spring, I began to learn who I was – and maybe
who I wasn't. It was a time of going within, a
frightening time in some ways, a time of change
and great mystery.

I learned to meditate. Slowly, I was learning to
take care of myself in a new way – a healthy way.

It had rained all that winter morning and the woods were saturated. Oh my, though! The colors in *"Nature's Palette"* were extraordinary. The better I felt, the more energy and light I saw – and the more my photos changed. The nature spirits shared their energy and light with me as I trusted my intuition – my heart. As I immersed myself ever more in nature, hiking became a walking meditation. As I meditated and walked, I felt more deeply and heard more clearly. I could feel the touch of the nature spirits on the side of my face and on my head, as a loving presence. For me, this was what the touch of the Divine felt like.

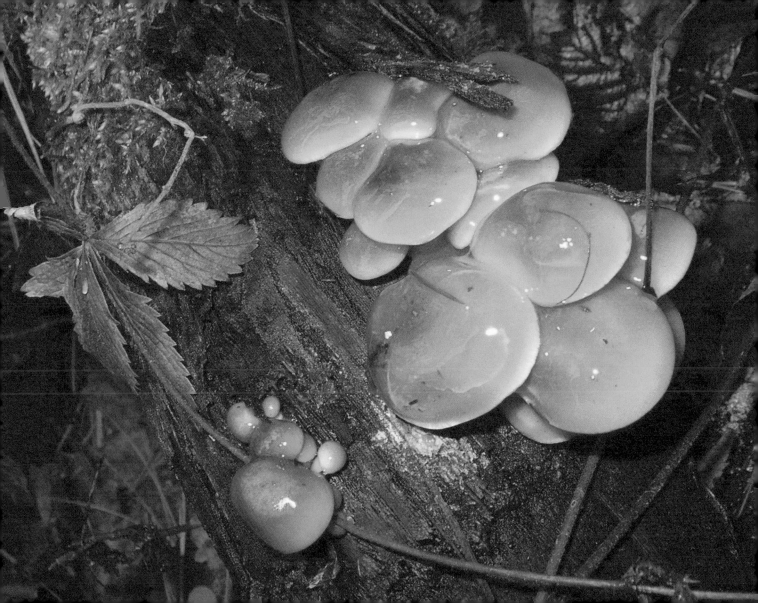

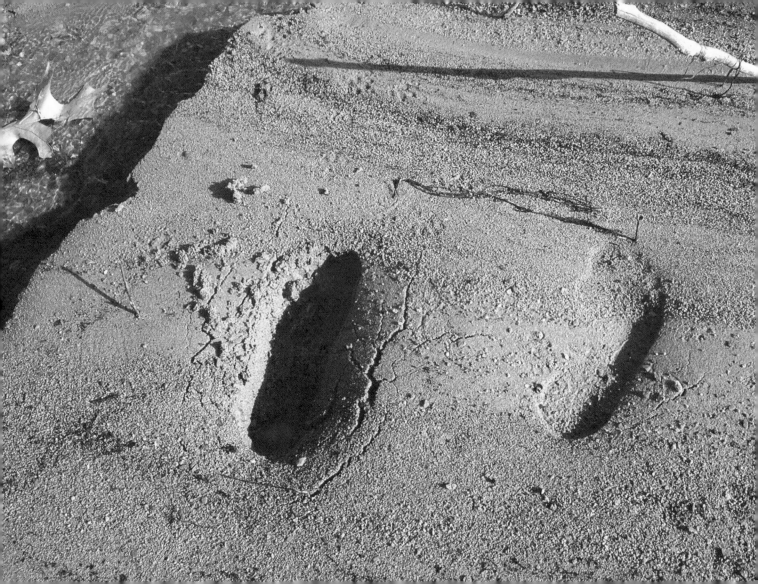

This was not an easy time. As I began to change deep inside, so did my relationships. Things that used to be okay – a gathering with friends to drink, for example – no longer felt right. This was a dying of sorts. As old friendships changed, I grieved their loss. I also began to isolate myself from any negative chatter around me.
I went to the woods to calm my spirit. I felt serene walking or sitting and just being. This was the place where I was being healed.

My images continually surprised me; the evidence of change was everywhere – inside me, in nature. This was my journey.

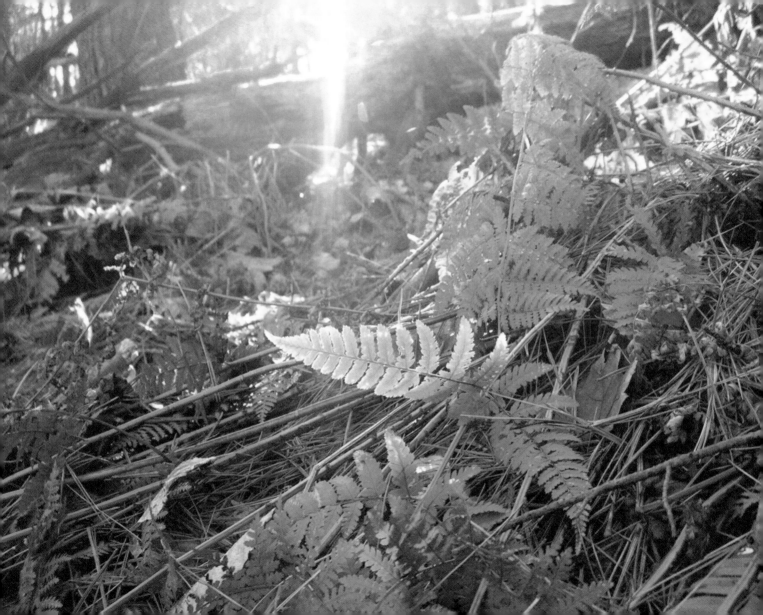

My photos held images I could not explain.
I kept following my heart. I tried to not
listen to my endless, fearful thoughts. The
more I did this, the more alive I felt.

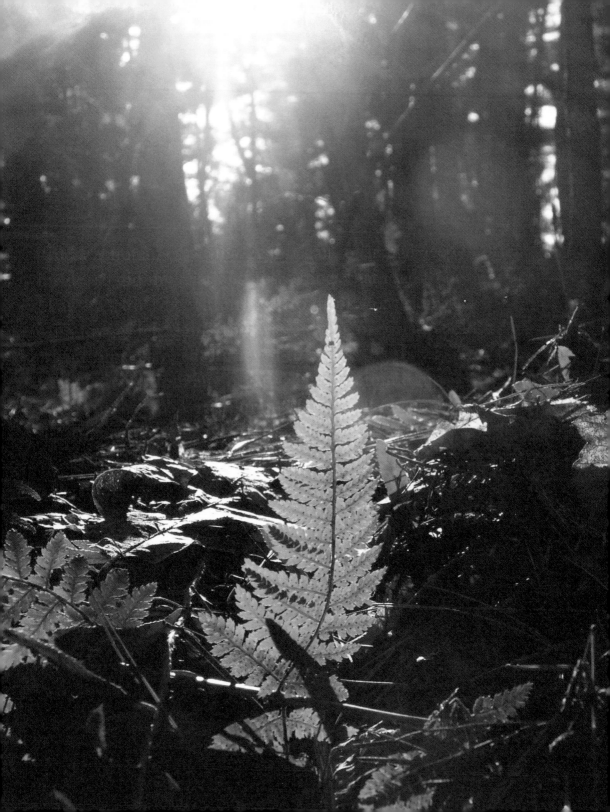

When I saw you, dear beautiful fern leaf,
standing in the afternoon light, my heart
felt full. As I embraced the earth you rose
from, I felt humbled by your beauty.

I became open, more *me*. As I walked in the woods, as I felt myself becoming new, I asked the Divine and my angels for a new name – a name that would fit me and the artist I had become.

During a walk in the woods, I heard that new name. It was *efy* –taken from eth-phatah meaning "be opened." I embraced *"efy."*

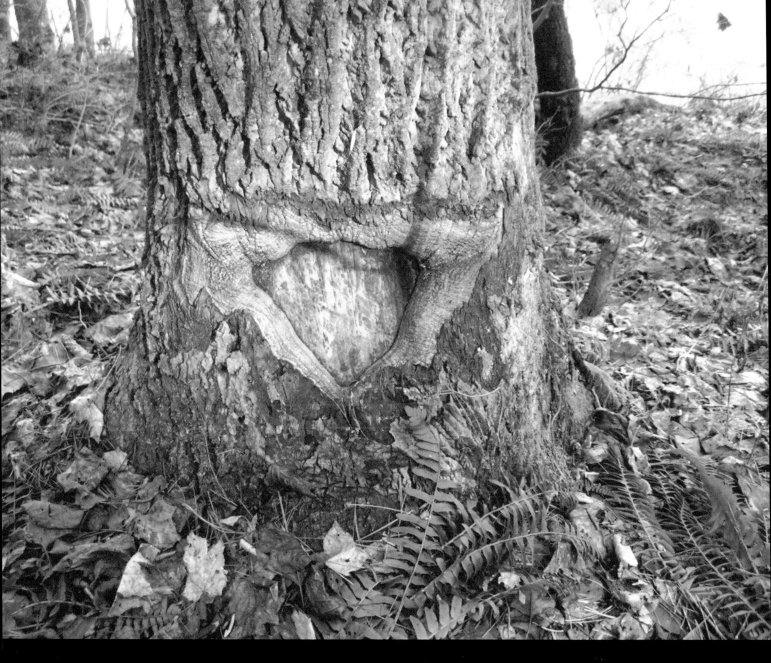

Open Heart

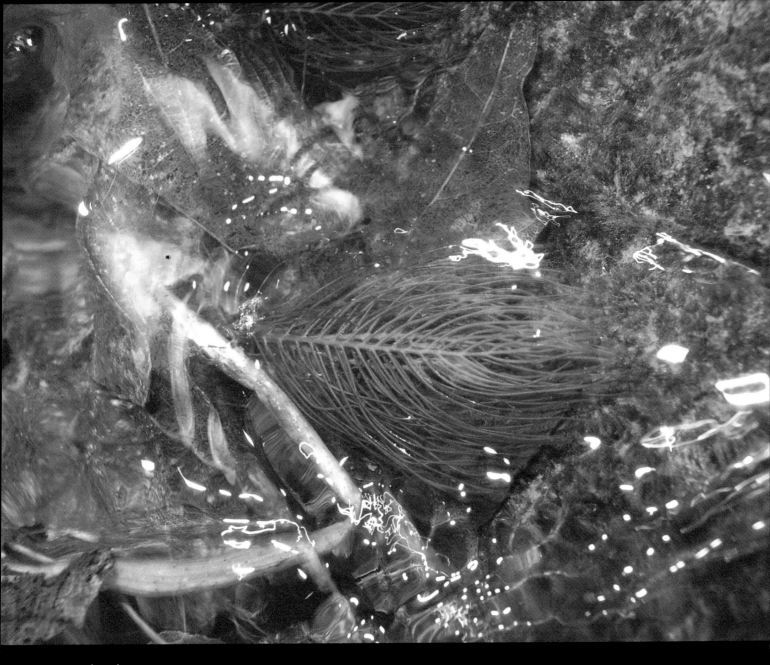

Gentle Flow

II. The Transition: The Heart Shatters

I'd never liked my birth name, never felt that "Lynda" fit me. I preferred nicknames like "Ike," or "Luc," short for Lucy. (Louise was my middle name.) It wasn't easy for my husband to call me "efy" or for my family of origin, or for my friends. I understood that it would be uncomfortable for people close to me to begin to use my new name, but I appreciated that they chose to honor my journey in this way.

I can't really explain how I felt. The old me did die – and then efy was born. The need to just be became more and more important. I was listening to the Divine. I could really be Me.

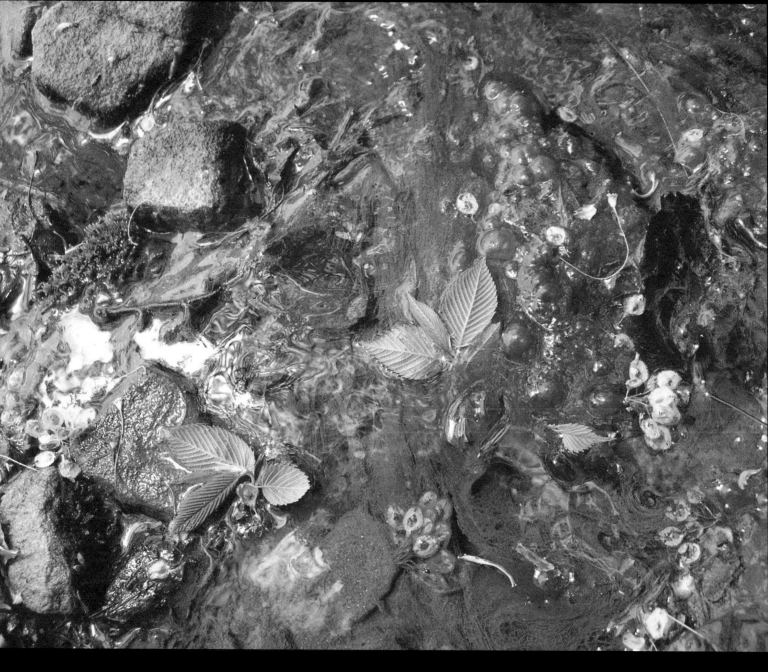

Discerning Waters

With the Divine, with my angels and nature spirits around me, I said YES to *me*, to efy.

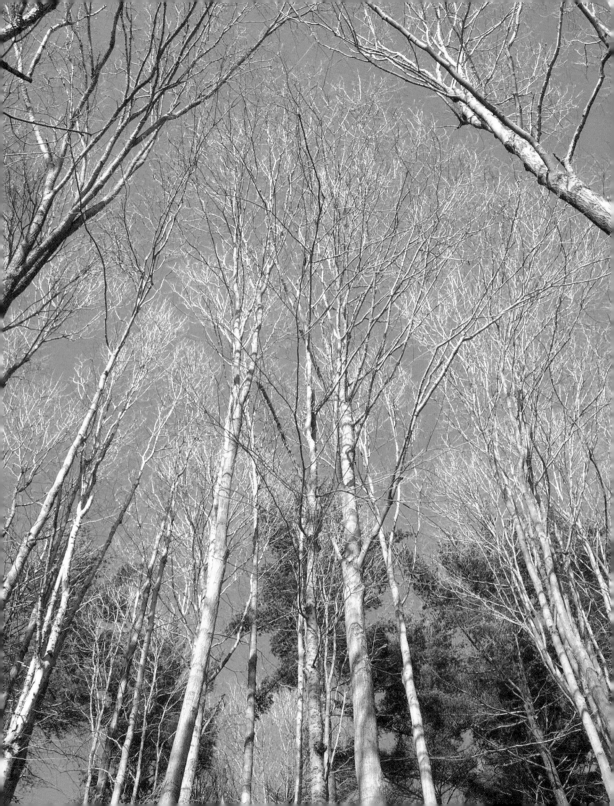

After one Reiki session, I felt "weird." Some fear was bubbling up. I went home, fell asleep, and had what I now can only explain as a "flashback." It took me months longer to recognize what the "flashback" meant and what it was about. As I tried to explain it to an understanding friend, she suggested I seek out a therapist to help me through this stage of my healing – and I'm thankful for her loving nudge. All along, my husband was supportive and as understanding as he could be. He was my best friend.

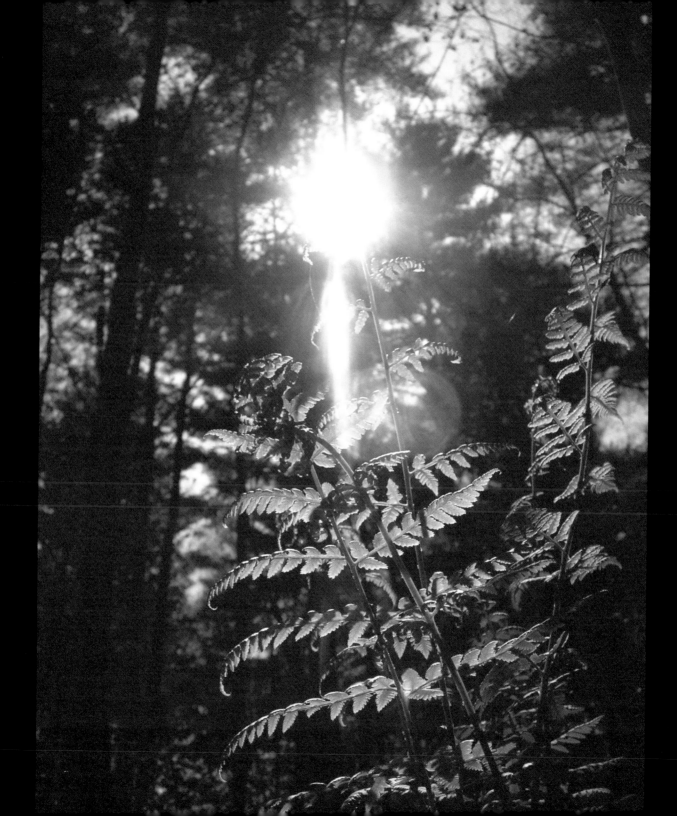

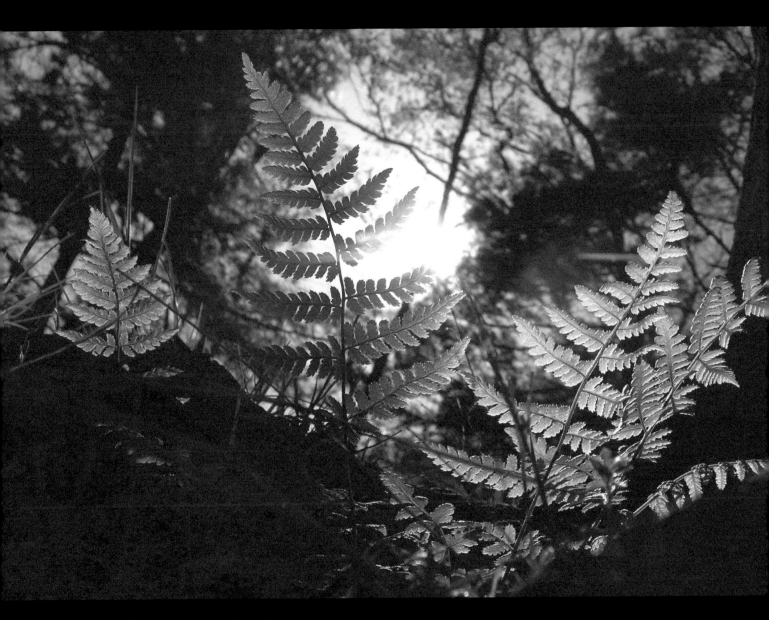

Inspiration

As I continued to receive Reiki and see a therapist about the flashbacks I was experiencing, they became more frequent and more frightening. As they intensified, symptoms from Lyme disease flared up. The shooting pains through my head and body returned. I felt like I was in a living hell and that I would be unable to get through it.

When I was able to say aloud to *myself* that I'd been sexually abused as a child, healing began. In the process of discussing my childhood trauma with a trusted therapist, I began to have more confidence that I could take care of myself. I feel we each must be responsible for our own life.

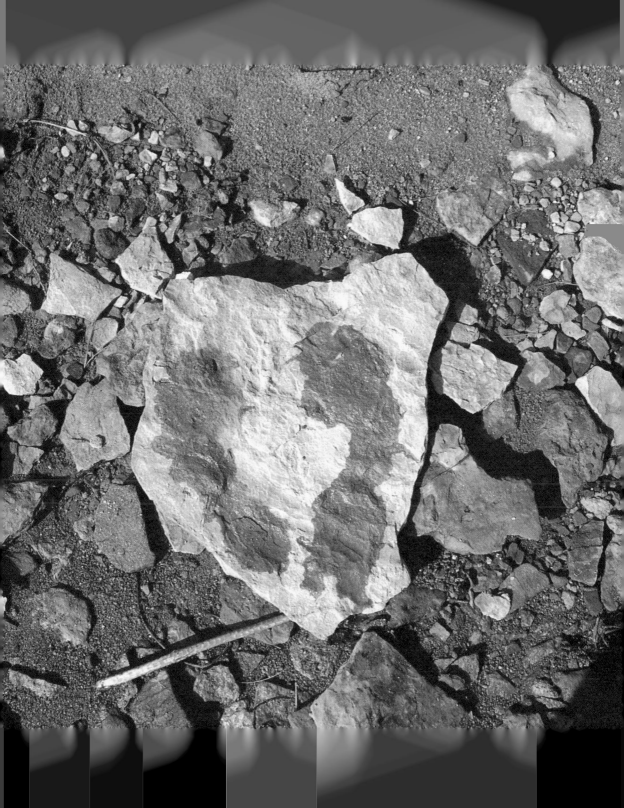

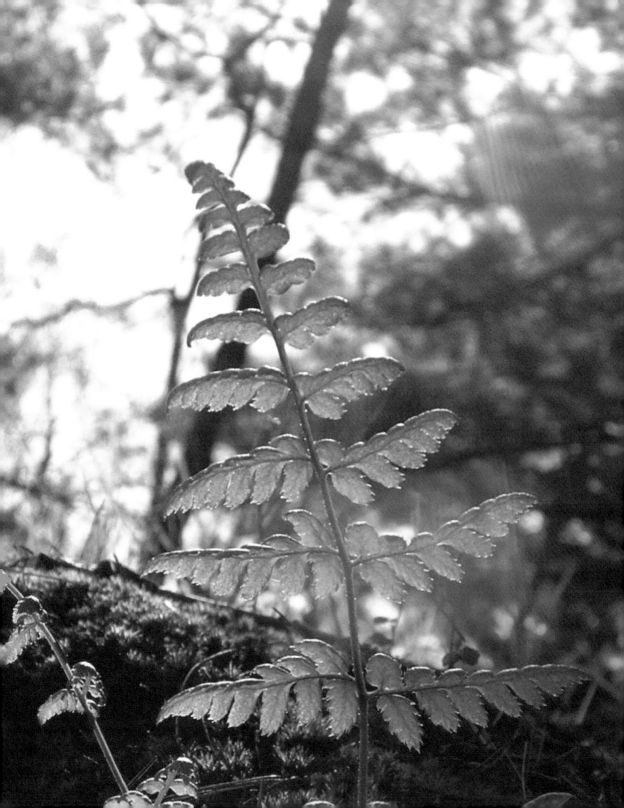

I was afraid to put down on paper the thoughts that rattled around in my head. But about nine months after my first visit to the Spring, I wrote in my journal:

I feel very deeply that my husband and I are not going to make it. It's not him. It's me — my heart is not in it. I don't want to hurt him or use him, but the only time I feel peaceful is at the lake and in the woods. The energy there beckons me and I feel stronger spiritually when I'm there — so much stronger. I feel like me.

But when I felt the pull to leave my marriage, I couldn't believe it. I didn't have many complaints. I felt grateful for my husband!

I heard a still small voice within me say, *Look at your marriage*. I grieved and grieved the day I realized my marriage was going to end. It felt like a death. I was afraid, very afraid. I usually walked in the woods at least once every day, but the day I realized I was going to leave my marriage – I walked and walked using my breath to calm my inner turmoil.

I was a mass of paradoxes and contradictions. I loved my husband – yet I was going to leave him. I contracted Lyme disease from ticks in the woods – yet the woods and the Spring were the only places I felt peaceful and at home with myself. That I so loved nature was, in itself, confusing and amazing. Nothing made much sense – except taking care of myself, listening to my inner voice (my intuition), going to the Spring, and walking in the woods. These were like mantras that I engaged every day as part of my healing.

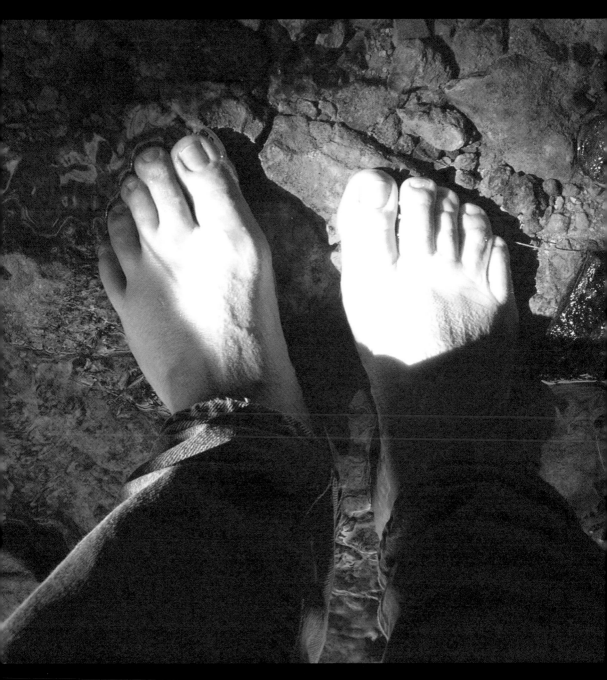

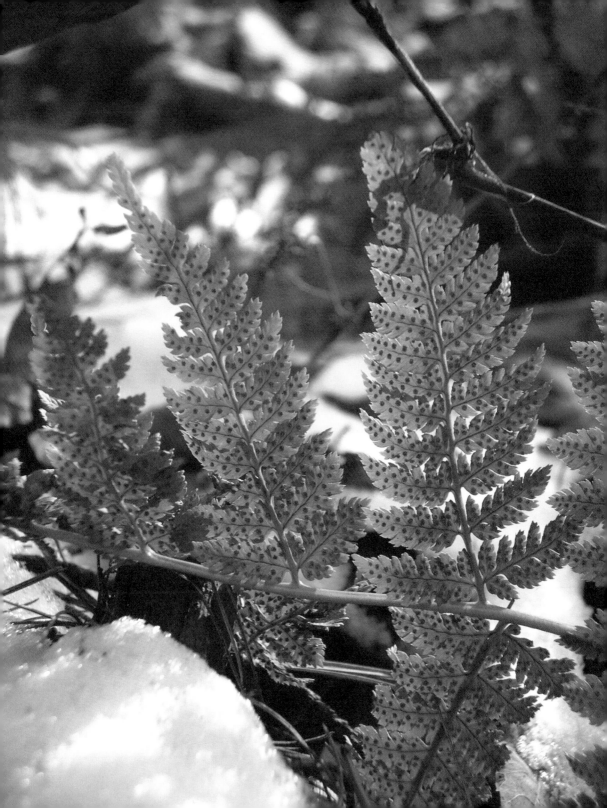

A hard realization was dawning on me as I found myself falling in love with nature and the Divine. I loved my husband and my son and they loved me. Yet, I was feeling drawn to a deeper and deeper call. Nature was healing me with every step I took on sacred ground. My true self, as efy, was being "opened."

I left my husband and my son who loved me – and I them. I confused them. I confused myself. They begged me not to leave.

The fear of being judged for my choices was very painful. But I also knew that if I did not deal with my own inner turmoil, I was of no use to anyone.

I moved – by myself – to a cabin on the lake near the Spring.

Every day, I pray for peace and understanding for all of us. I hope that my husband will be able to love me for who I am and to be my friend. These are big things to ask of him. I'm walking every day — sometimes twice — just trying to get through.

I look back now and believe I received a call from the Divine to change my life, to become who I really was. The call was loud and clear: Change your life. And the call felt right.

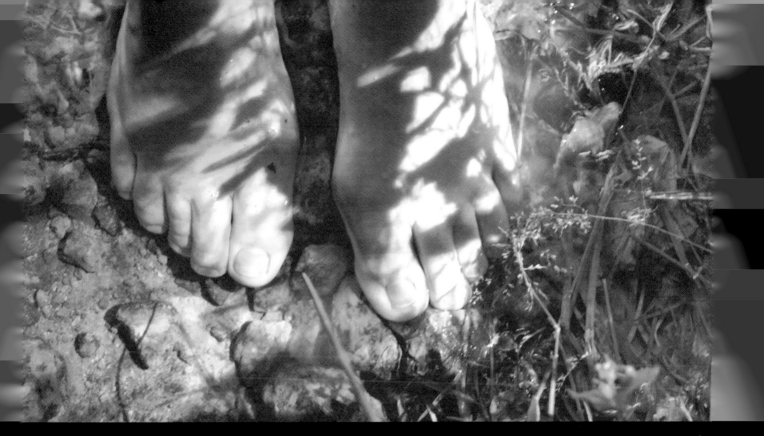

Forgive

My tears are sweet this night as they pass over my lips.

Will this grief ever unleash my soul – must this struggle be?

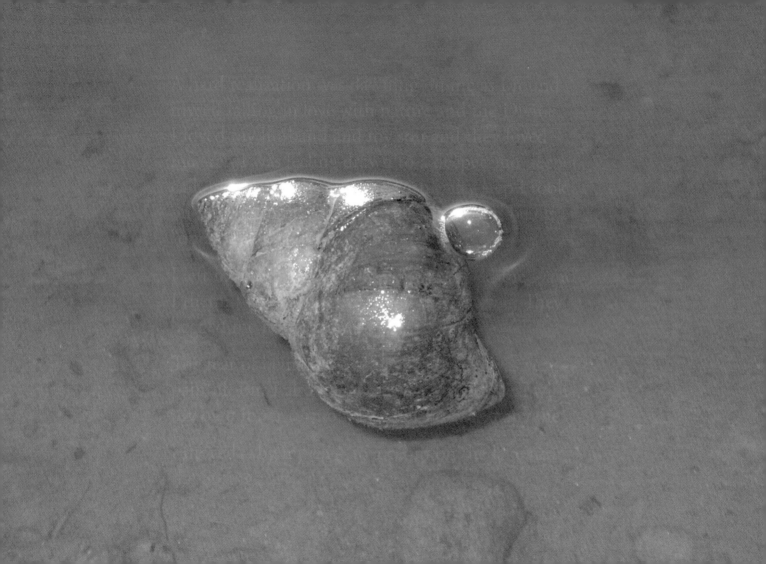

As difficult as this time was for me and
for my family, I felt divinely guided as
I began a year of self-isolation. I lived
simply. Many hours of reflective prayer
and the love of supportive friends got me
through. Nature kept inviting me in.

Alone in the cabin, I had flashbacks. I was afraid.
I didn't know if I could survive this painful time.
Yet, I knew this was about trusting the Divine
and releasing past hurts. The more I released
those past hurts, the better I felt.

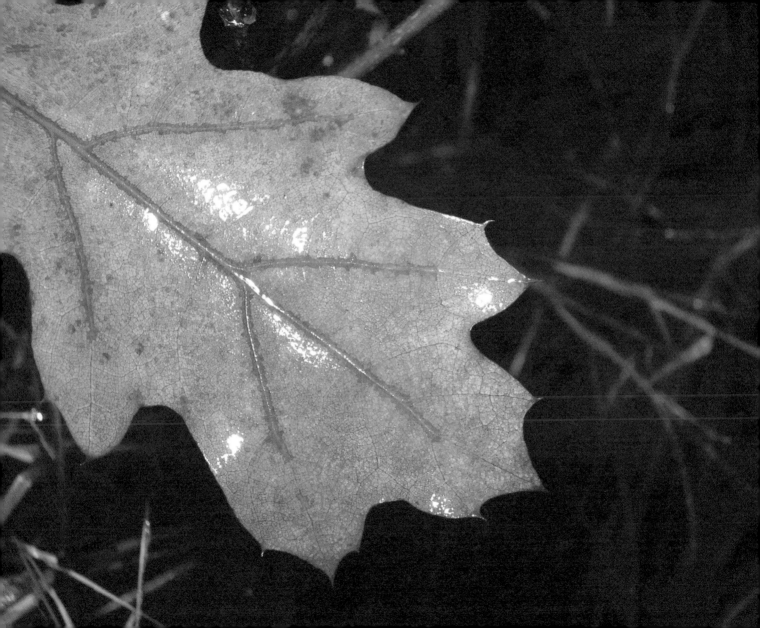

I saw your painting this morning. Everywhere I looked you, the Divine, had been there. My heart was in awe — beauty all around me, sunlight streaming through the trees, the color of leaves so vibrant — so full of your love. May I never be blind to you and your love!

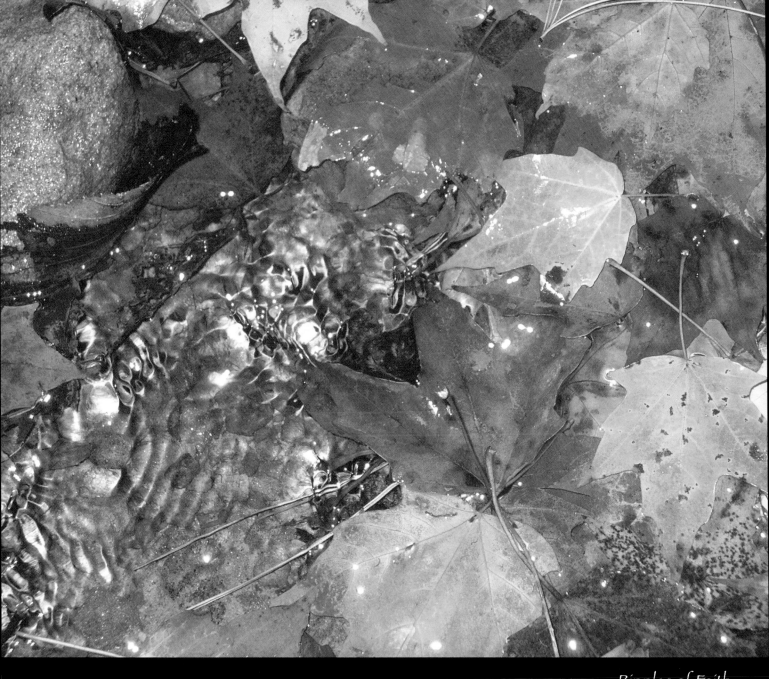

Ripples of Faith

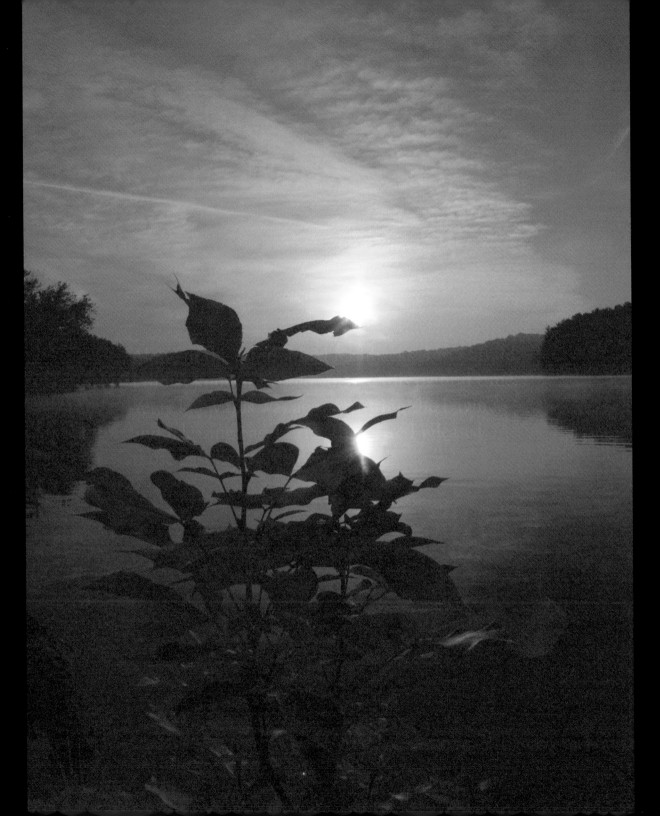

Are you within me – speaking the truth when I can't?

Please don't let go as my arms are tired and I can't hold on much longer. Your gentleness is warm and loving –

Please don't let go!

love, efy

I'd always wanted to have a photography business, but I was never clear on how I'd do it or what I would specialize in. At this point I wasn't aware that a business was even in my future. I was taking photographs for myself, for the simple joy it gave me.

My images continued to amaze me, gift me, heal me. As I hiked around the woods that first year in my cabin, I became clear about the work I was being asked to do. I felt ready to begin living *my* truth, *my* integrity, *my* awe. Things change in the woods at every season, from year to year. What I photographed last year at this time was no longer there. So I found an intensity in each moment and I focused on being in that moment so I would miss none of it. I saturated myself in the newness.

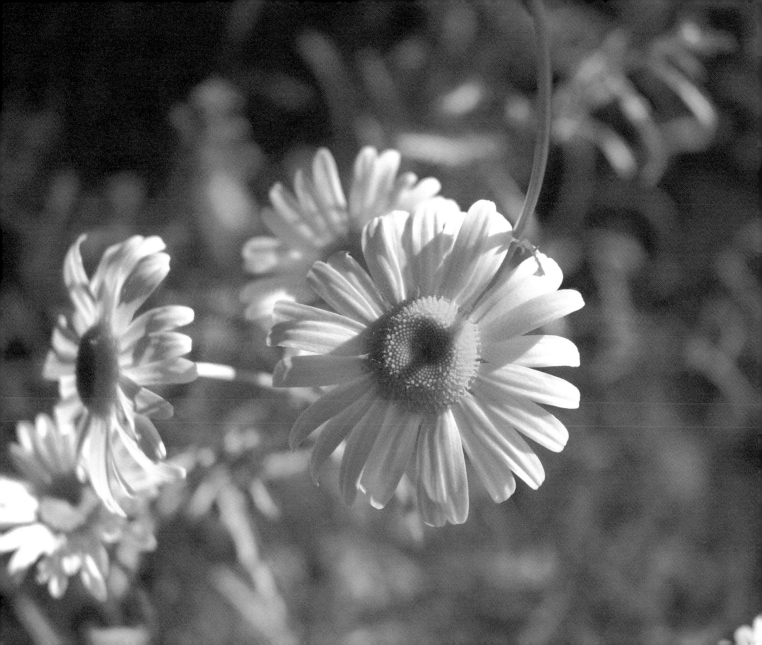

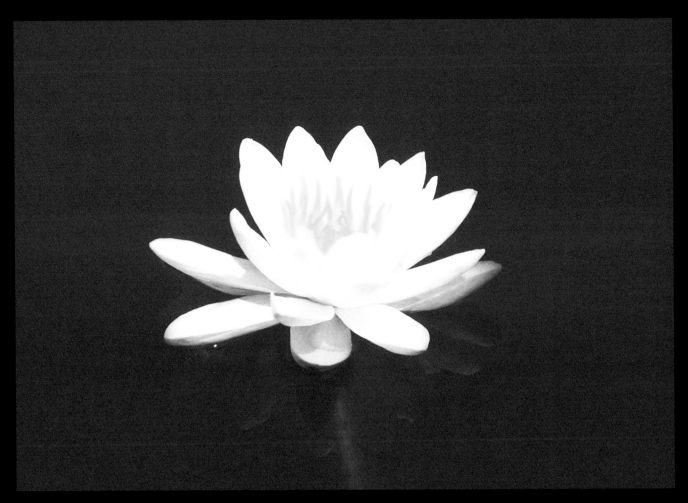

Solemn Lotus

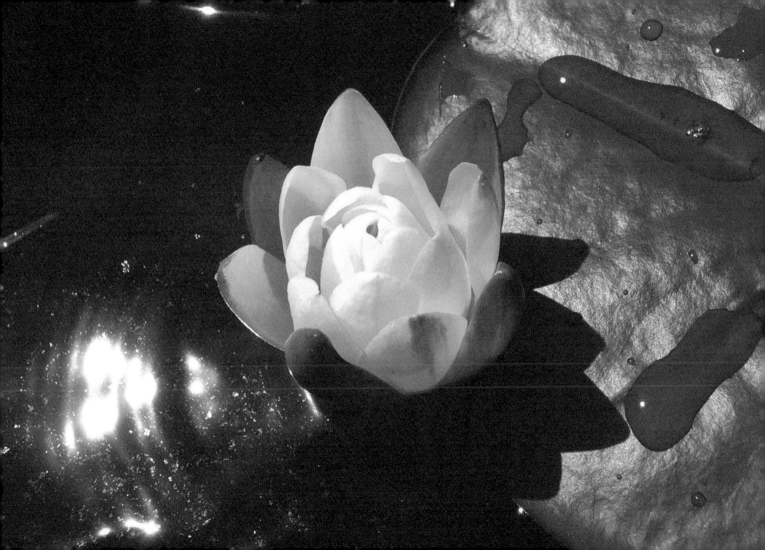

I feel as though I have been opened and my journey for now is to share what I see and feel and capture with my camera. This is my work – this is where my heart is leading – this is efy's purpose.

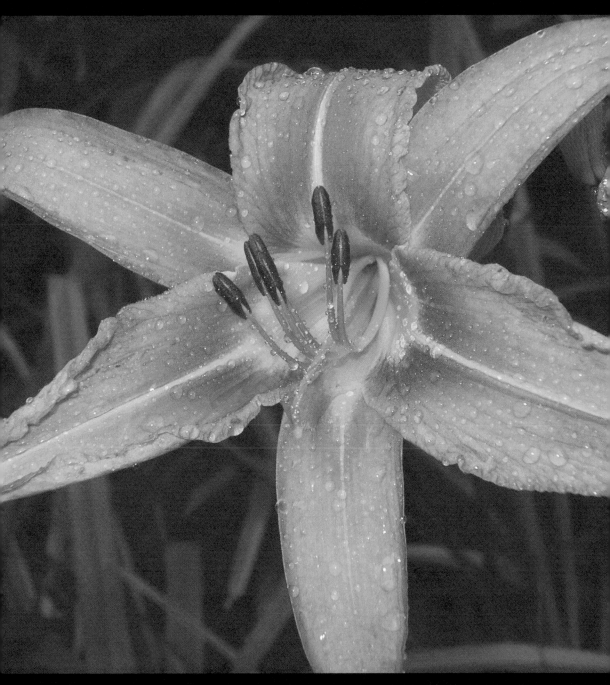

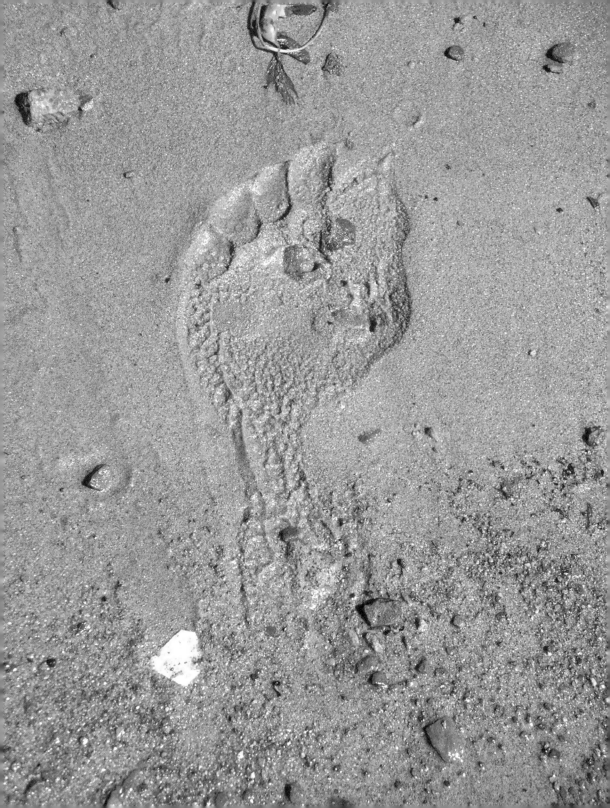

Evidence of the Holy One

Is everywhere I look
Under my feet
My feet in all their amazing ability
The leaves in all their amazing color
The water in all its clarity
The stones, their gentle way of holding me

Why do I look at fire and see my soul?
A small flame striving to be like the Full Flame
Like the vine and branches
My soul dances because the Holy One dances

I am as intricate as the fern leaf, all those
Parts of me that hang on, that shine, that
Drip with love

Angel wings, rivers of light,
The flow of my life, moving, changing
Blessed, blessed, blessed

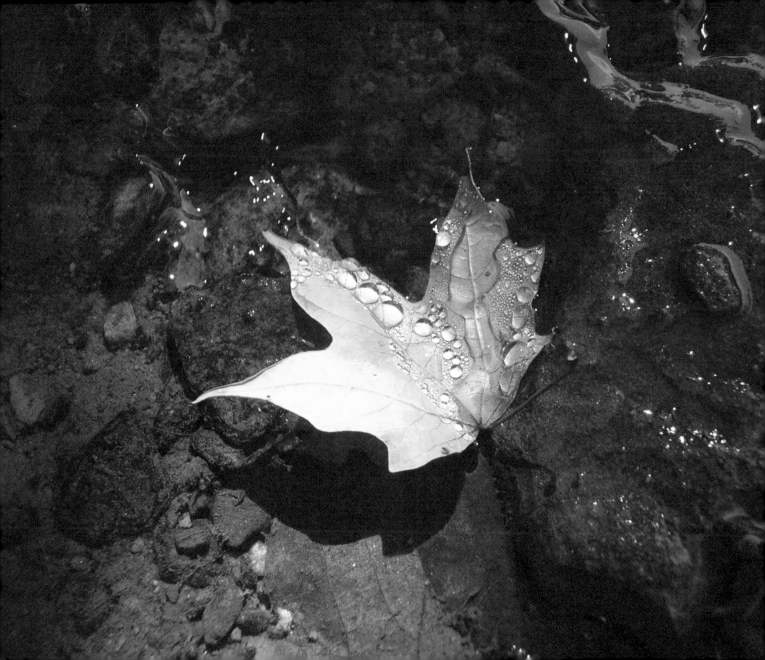

I see perfection.

I wonder if it sees me

If Light Guides are all around us
Why do I so often worry?

My soul and its little light
Forgetting that it is not other
Than Big Light

Asking us to see what is
And what is not

Sometimes I don't see
Sometimes I do.

When I would leave the woods to head back to my cabin, my family was not there. Each time, it surprised me. I kept thinking, How could this be?

How could I feel at home living in the middle of the woods – all alone – without them?

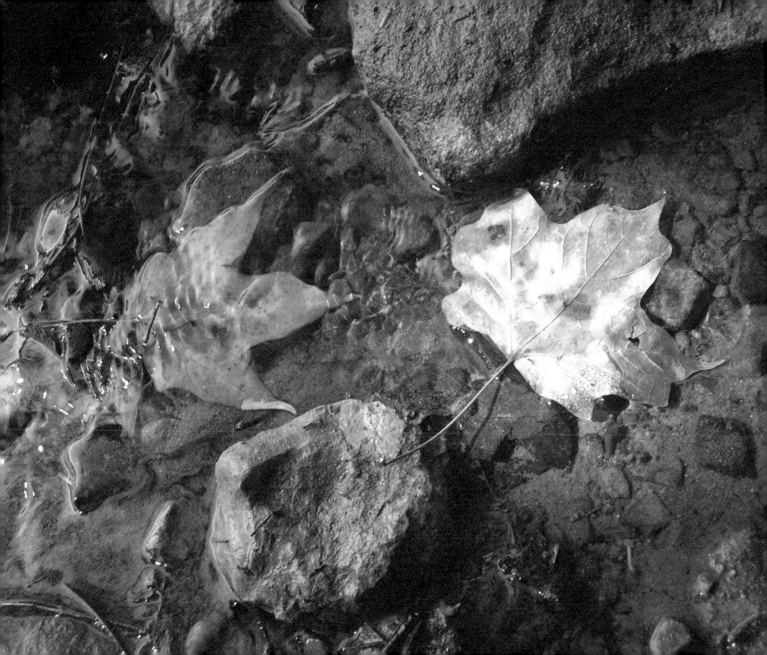

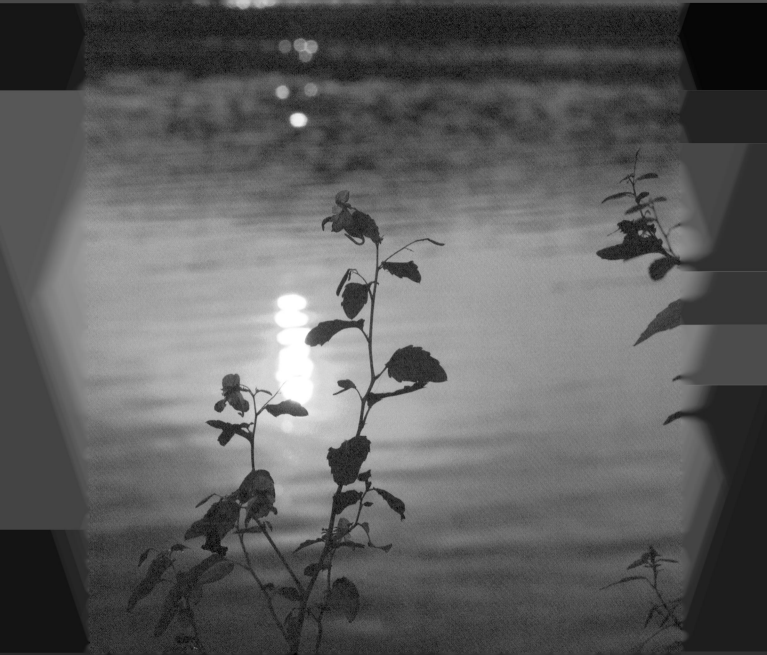

I left all that was safe and secure, the people
who had nurtured me and loved me for so
long – who had loved me more than I could
put into words. I grieved very deeply.

Yet, my soul would not let me live what I no longer was. I had been dying – inside and out. I couldn't ignore what my body and soul were telling me. What a strange realization it was.

At times, I would become afraid of the quiet in the cabin in the woods at night – but then I understood that those were the times I would learn to truly know myself. I would listen to the Divine. In the end I would come to relish the quiet of my own isolation. I would face my fears and put them to rest. I became stronger. And for that, I thank Godde!*

*I love this spelling of the word we use for the Divine of all. It combines God and Goddess and reminds me that the Divine is both male and female – or maybe neither.

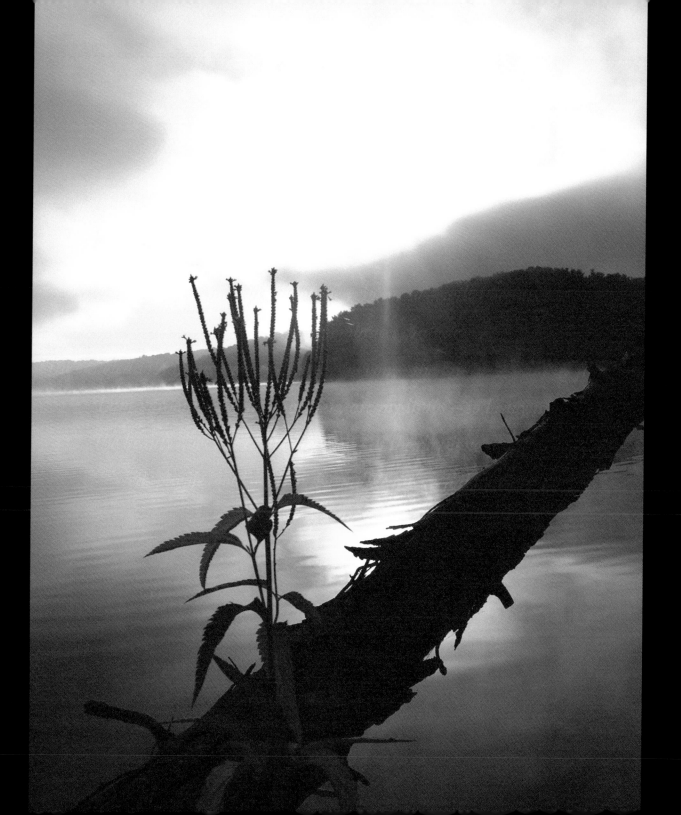

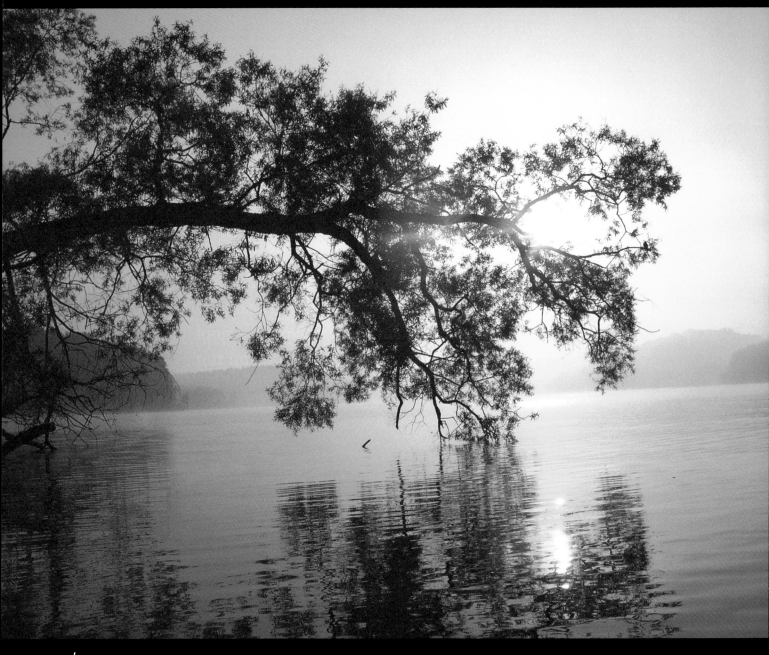

Solace Gaze

I wrote this in my journal while thinking of my son:

I hope you can still love and accept me. I want to be happy – I want you to be happy. I did not want to hurt you. I did not leave your Dad for anyone – for anyone – but myself. I am finally beginning to be happy. I love you.

Over and over I would say to myself *I am sorry, please forgive me, I love you.*

This near isolation was vitally important for me. I needed to face my fears, alone.

On a very cold day along a river, I felt
Spirit flowing. Then, in the river, I saw the
angelic presence woven into the waters.

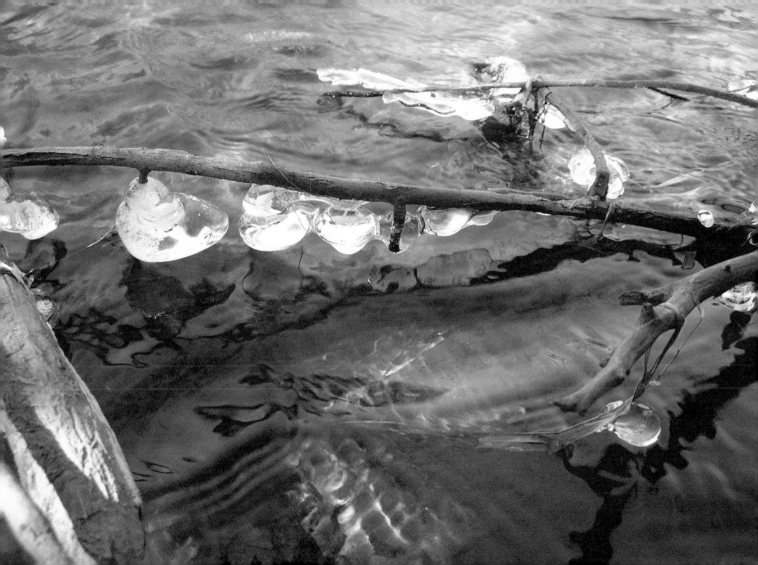

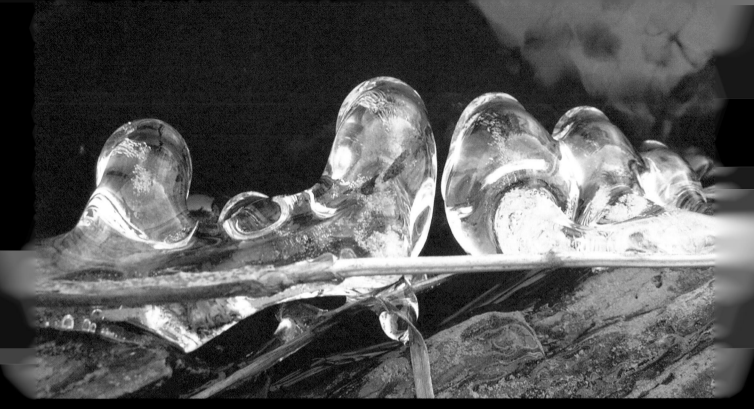

ce Birds

All day I felt the presence of the Divine. I lay on the bank to get a closer look at this image.

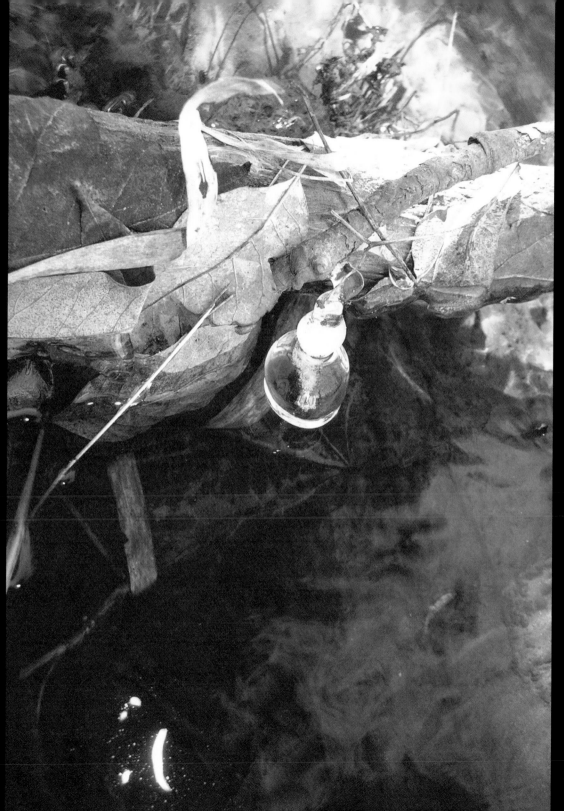

Peace Bird

The quiet depths of life grip me so – will I breathe?

My mind embraces solitude.

The tangled vibrations seem endless – Abwoon – the Divine – vibrates from within.

I am without strength – so heavy are my limbs – so heavy is my heart.

The beauty does not escape my eyes – as the day-long sun bids goodbye –

red, purple, gold – all so warm like an eternal flame in the sky.

Peace

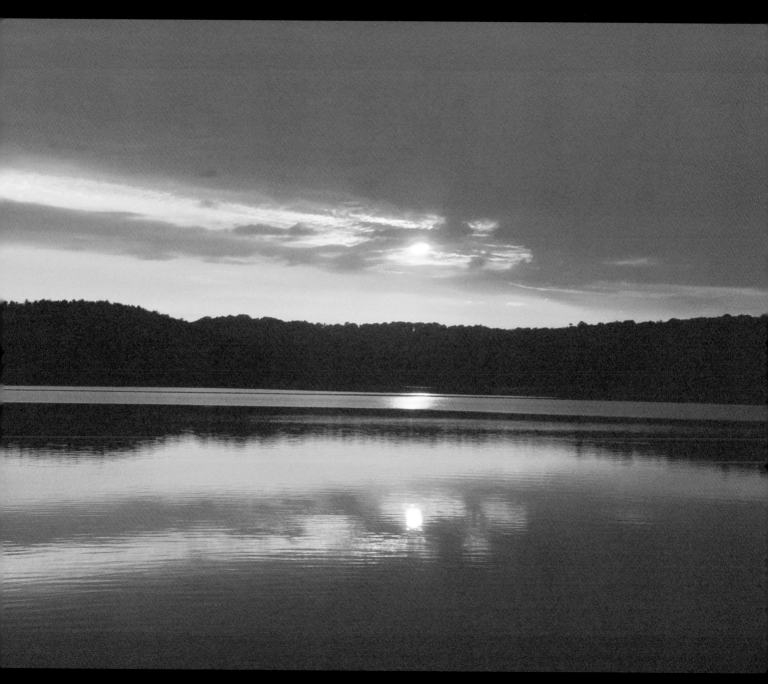

Eternal Sky

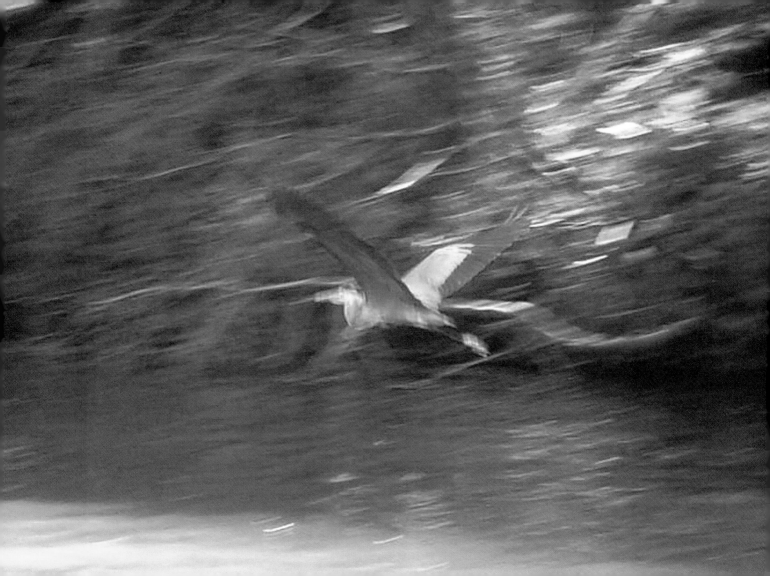

III. The Healing: Gift of Clarity

If I were a Heron, I would spread my wings out wide!
Soaring – soaring to the sky.
Ah freedom – so sweet.
Let me be free – oh let me be free.

Alone at the cabin, I began my love
affair with the Great Blue Heron.

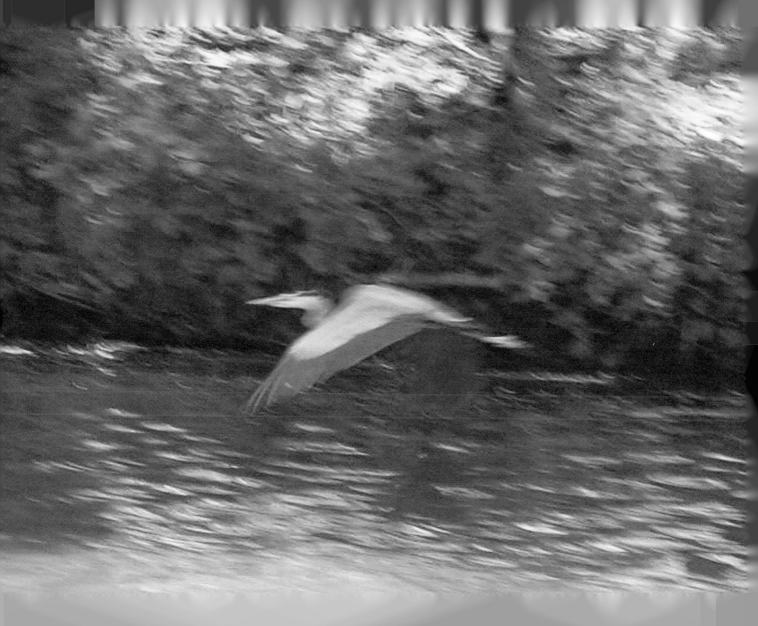

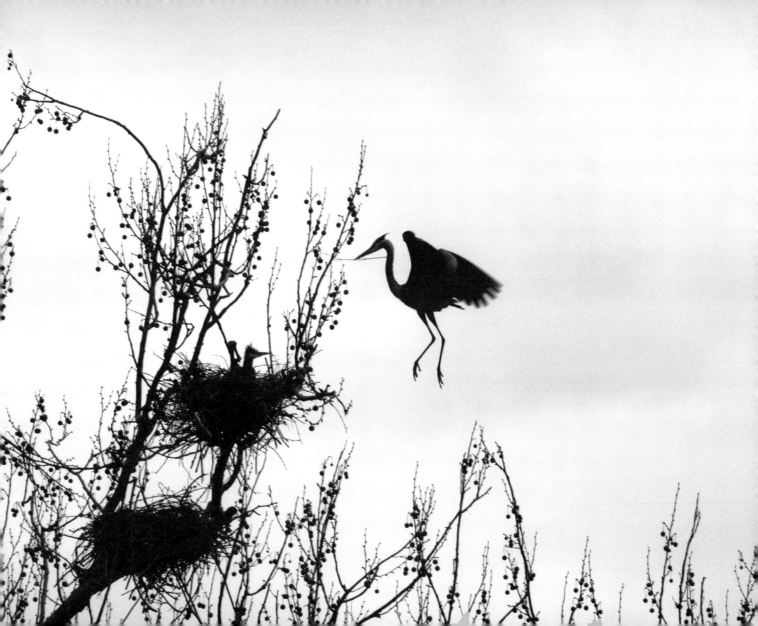

I talked to the herons and they didn't fly away when I approached and spoke. Instead, they posed for me and played tag with me. Their grace is beautiful.

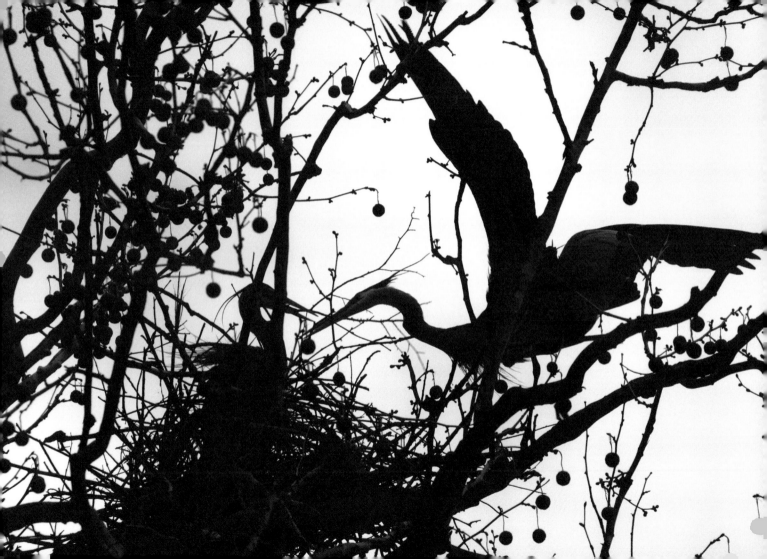

The love that they share together melts my heart and bubbles my emotions to the surface. I was also drawn to a nearby heronry, where I watched them build a nest and prepare for their young. Blessed Be!

Ah – as you cuddled and snuggled I could feel your love and then with your beautifully feathered bodies you formed a heart. I love you Heron!

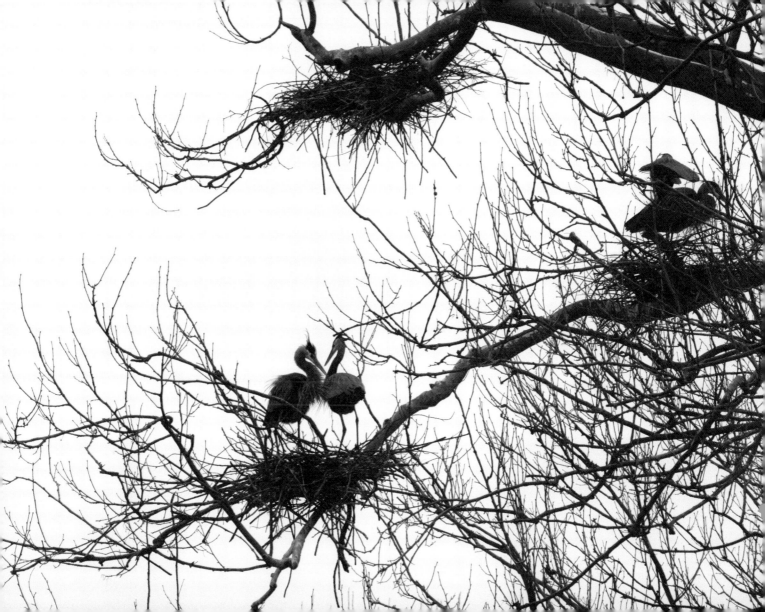

Where are you headed, dear one? Oh the journey at times seems so surreal. Where are you headed? Won't you please grace me with your strong wings? I want to fly with you.

Daily, I'm surrounded by the Divine and by angels, and I feel blessed. I feel the love and energy of the universe when Spirit appears in my images.

I bought a kayak and more of the natural world opened to me.
Today is a Gift.

As I float along your surface

I feel as though I am one with you.

I am – as I embrace and feel your presence.

The stillness of this morning is beyond words.

I have only feelings.

At One

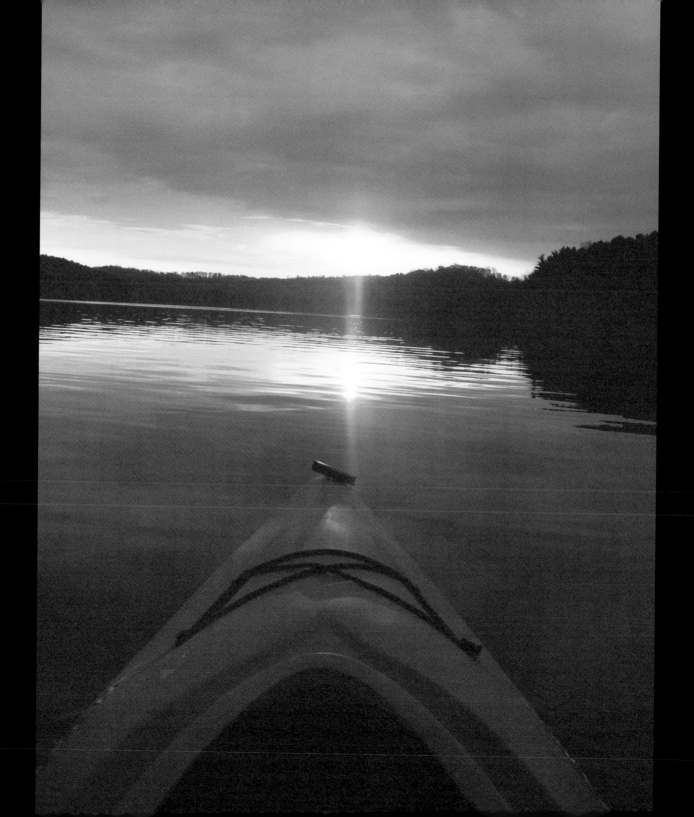

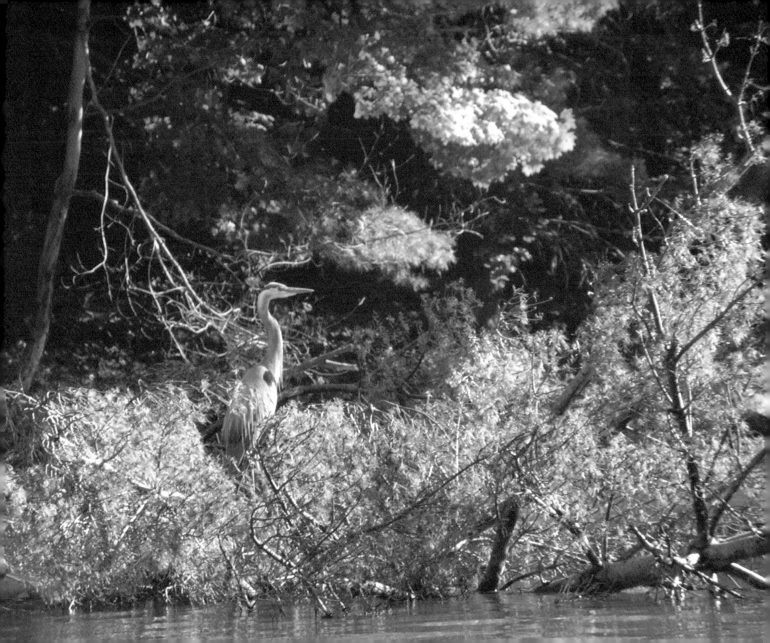

Wait – I have a song in my heart –

Let it sing as though it will never end

As though no one is listening.

Don't be afraid to be heard.

They may like your song!

Oh but the doubt –

I would often shed my shoes and
walk barefoot as I allowed Godde
to open me and my intuition.

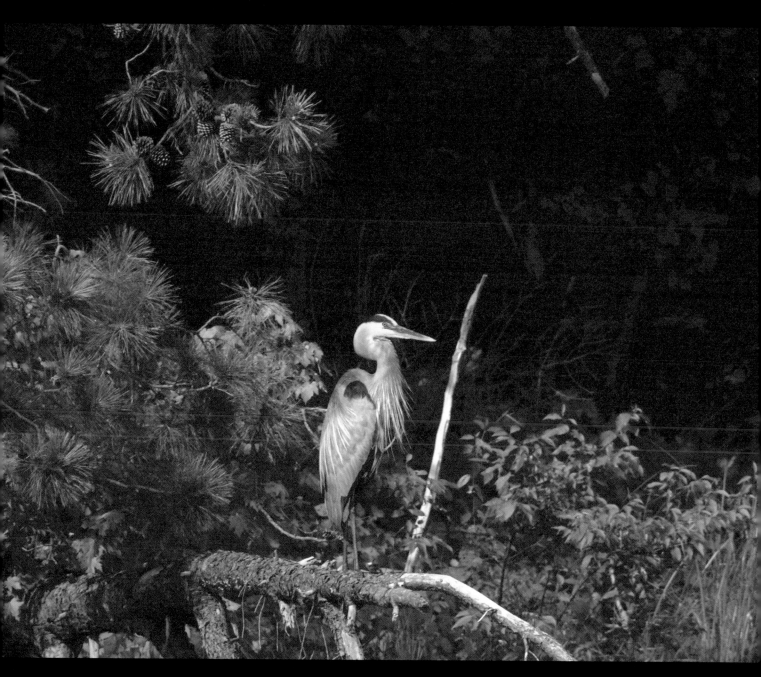

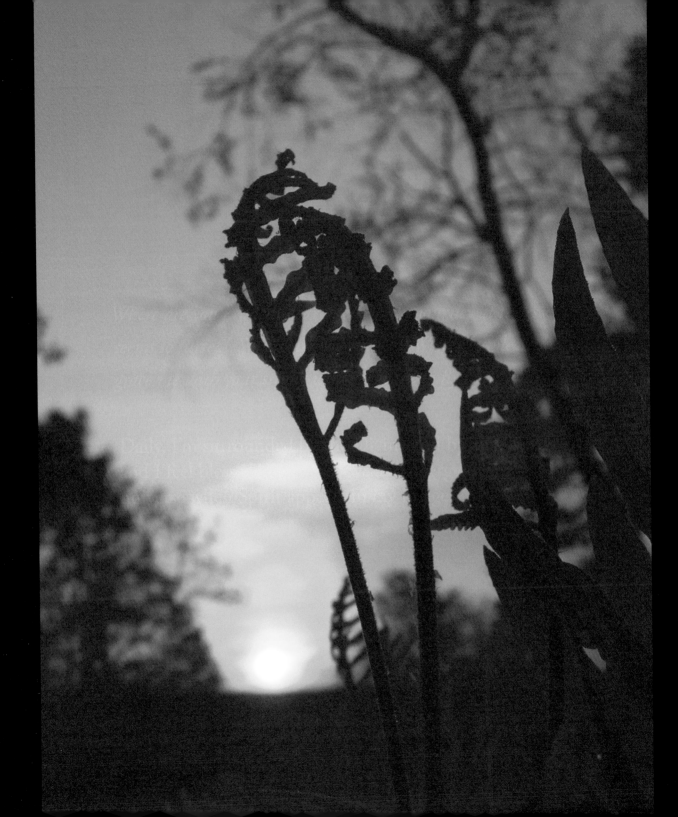

Whenever I walked in the woods I'd feel the energy from my feet all the way up to my head and out to my hands holding my camera. When I saw something I wanted to photograph, I'd feel a vibration and a loving energy. Almost before I could ask nature for permission to take a photo, permission would be granted – and that would give me more energy. I loved it! I'd get as close as I could, down on my hands and knees, embracing the ground, so that I could be one with the nature photo I was taking. I had a relationship with the natural world that was growing and deepening and I loved it – and it was loving me back.

As I was pulling my kayak up to land one evening, I noticed some very beautiful ferns. Often, I'd feel a nudge in my soul from a fern as I walked by. But that evening, the fern whispered directly to me, *"Come back tomorrow morning and take my picture!"*

I left my cameras out that night and as the sun came up the next morning, I was there with the ferns. Again I knelt and was moved and grateful for the images that beautiful morning. It was not unusual for me to hear guidance from nature or the Divine. And somehow, it was not just a fern! Somehow. I can't explain it.

I named this photo "eth-phatah!" Be open. How beautiful, oh how beautiful. This is the grace that fills my heart and soul.

eth-phatah

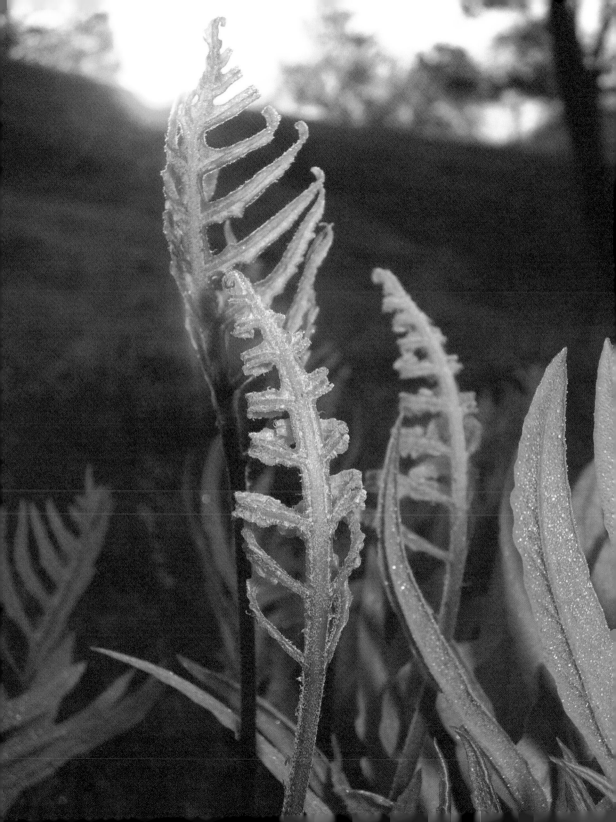

Other times I saw a great shot but I
didn't feel the connection, the energy,
the vibration. I didn't feel it in my heart.
I had no nudge, so I didn't take the shot.

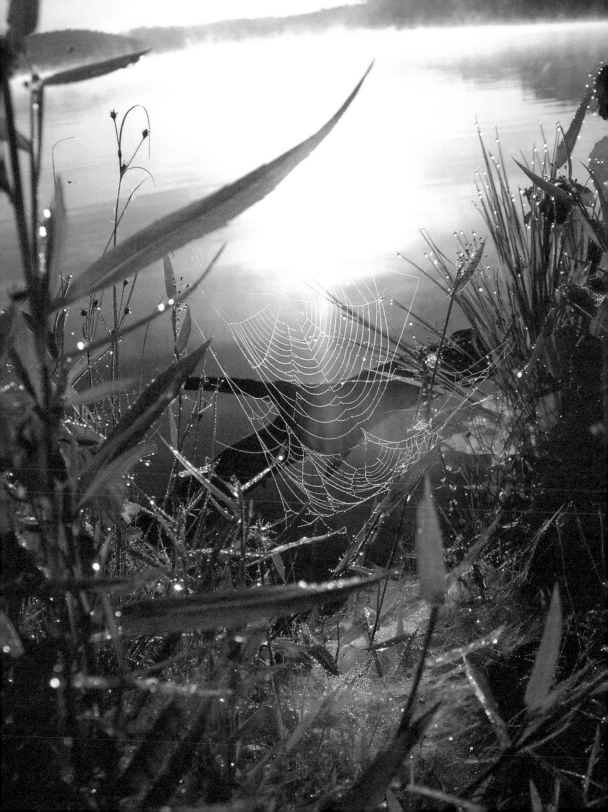

Mother Earth was giving me back my health, and I kept going back for more. I wasn't comfortable if, for some reason, I had to leave the woods or my cabin. I'd miss the feeling of being "home." Now, I finally feel at home in myself, wherever I am, because I'm living in my truth.

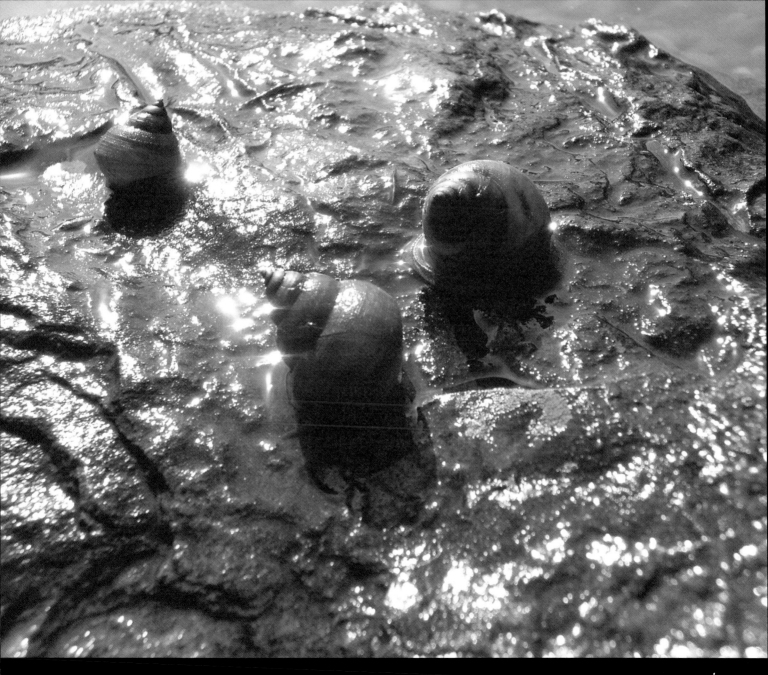

Peace Within

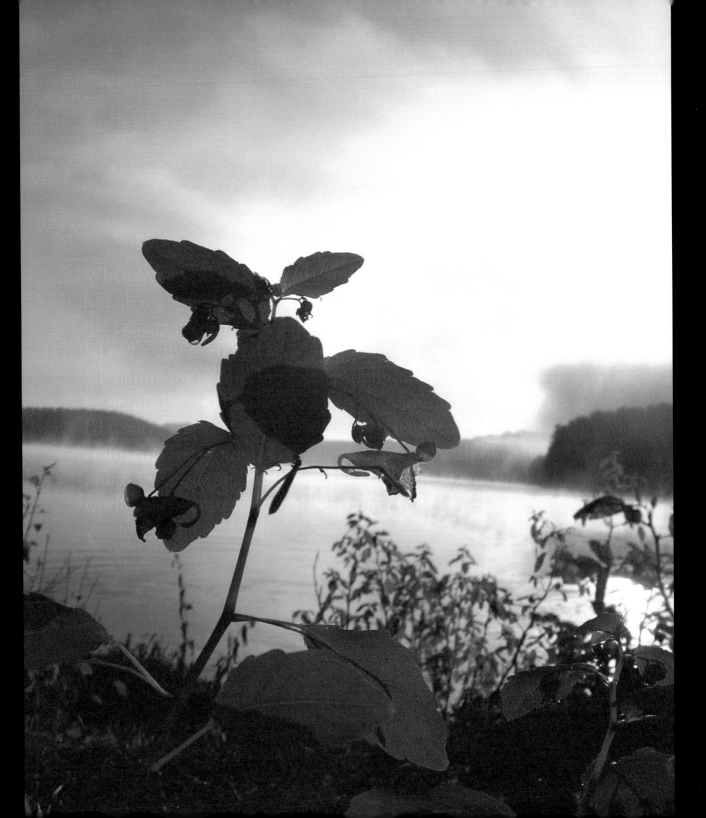

I am no longer afraid of the silence.

My heart is at peace and I am listening, feeling,

seeing Spirit in all.

The Heron was at the water's edge this crisp morning – in the far cove.

He lingered as I – we – spent that time being present to one another.

My journey has brought me here to this place – to this peace.

Finding truth and clarity was not – and is not – easy. But that was my journey. I learned that there would be a dip – okay, sometimes several dips – before a plateau would signal that I was ready for deeper healing.

My next healing was to say out loud that I was gay. I talked openly and honestly with my ex-husband and son about it. They could not understand, but they were loving and accepting.

I came out to family and friends. I didn't know if I could trust the Divine in this, if I could even trust myself. So I just trusted. I knew that if I didn't get right with myself, I could never be right with anyone else.

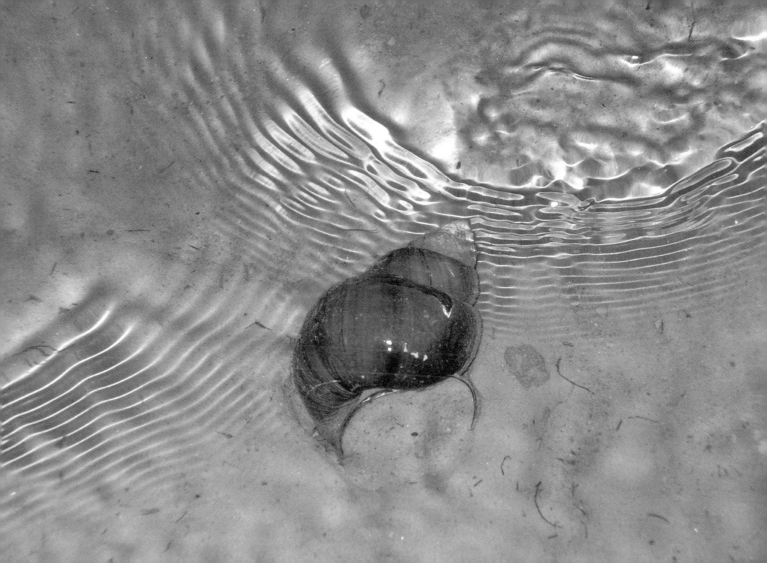

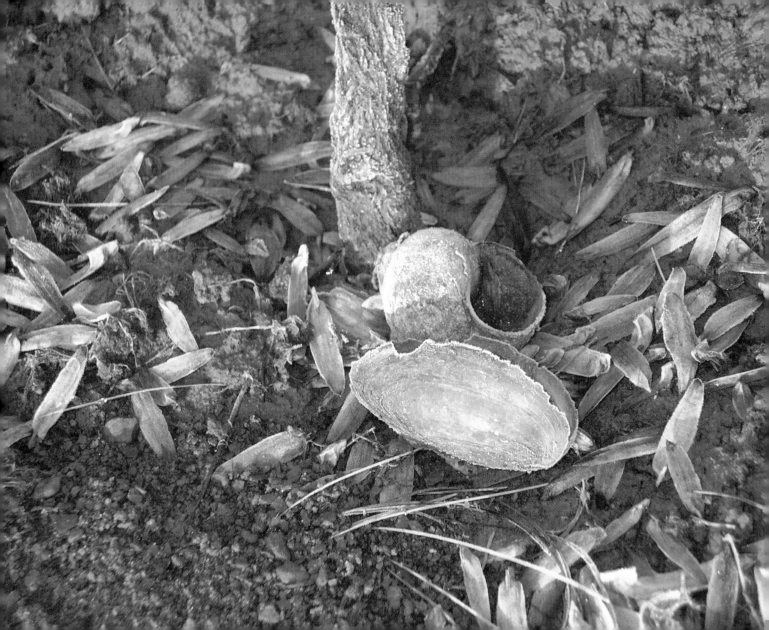

I was grateful to finally figure out who I was. I had become completely honest with myself. I healed in my own time, as my own journey directed. It wasn't as simple as saying "I want to heal myself." I had a lot of work to do, and that is the work that helped heal me. My first step was to become present to my own life. Then I became honest and embraced my own truth. When I embraced truth, more came to me. Healing was a continuous process – and it arrived with a new fear: being judged.

I got to the point that I trusted no matter what. I trusted that I'd be protected in the love of the Divine, who started me on this journey. Finally, I listened to the still small voice that loved me through it all. If we listen long enough, listening becomes comfortable.

This is where I'm filled with grace. I want to walk in your grace. Please let me walk in your grace.

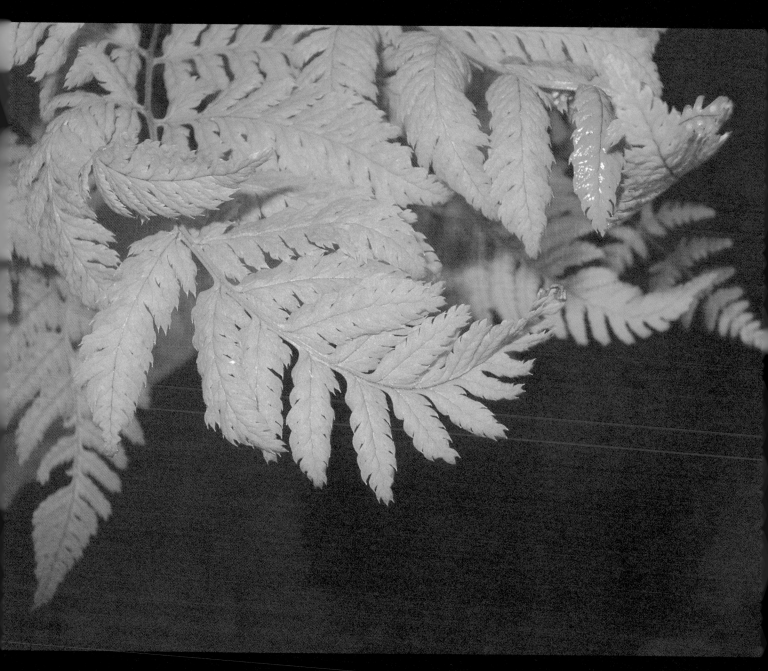

Frond Beauty

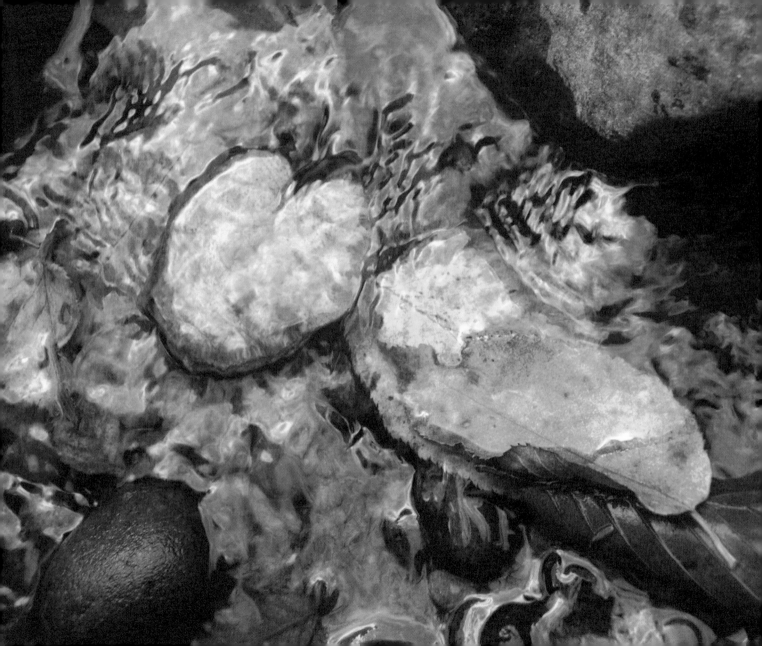

Oh how you touched my heart with a forever love.
I will walk in this grace, filled with gratitude.

Life brought me a new love, a feeling I had never felt before. I loved her from deep within my soul and heart. And though I hoped our love would last forever, it did not. It was with a heavy and grieving heart that I let her go.

Yet, I'm so happy I said "yes." *Yes* to new love in my life . . . yes to the unknown … yes even to the darkness, for I've learned that being completely vulnerable blesses me, makes me humble. As I walk the path of life, I am presented with what I need at just the right time. I feel blessed, I feel thankful.

This love was part of my path too, part of my journey, ultimately part of my healing. Not that I wasn't overwhelmed with tremendous grief . . . again. A shattering of my heart, again. Yet the relationship taught me so much more about love and about myself. I healed more deeply. How can I not be grateful? It was BEAUTIFUL, in every way! What a grace-filled time. The Divine continues to amaze me as my life unfolds in mystery. All I need do is show up, trust, and say "Yes" and "Thank you"!

I feel like I'm dancing with the Divine.

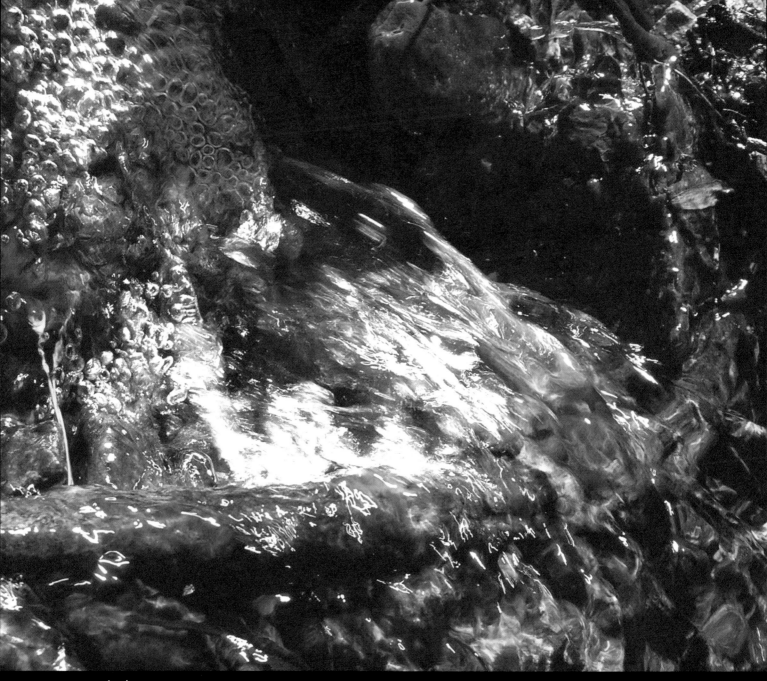

Sacred Play

Dancing with the Divine

In the stillness of this night,
I was danced by the Divine!
We danced slowly and in rhythm with one another.
Under the moonlit sky for a time,
leaving only one set of footprints in the snow.
As my body moved in your vibration and my rhythm.
I felt you, the Divine, in every step and in every breath I took.
I felt you linger for a time
my limbs feeling tired as my body bows to sleep.
Please stay for a while as I give thanks
for this grace-filled day.
For it is with you that I
have found my truth.

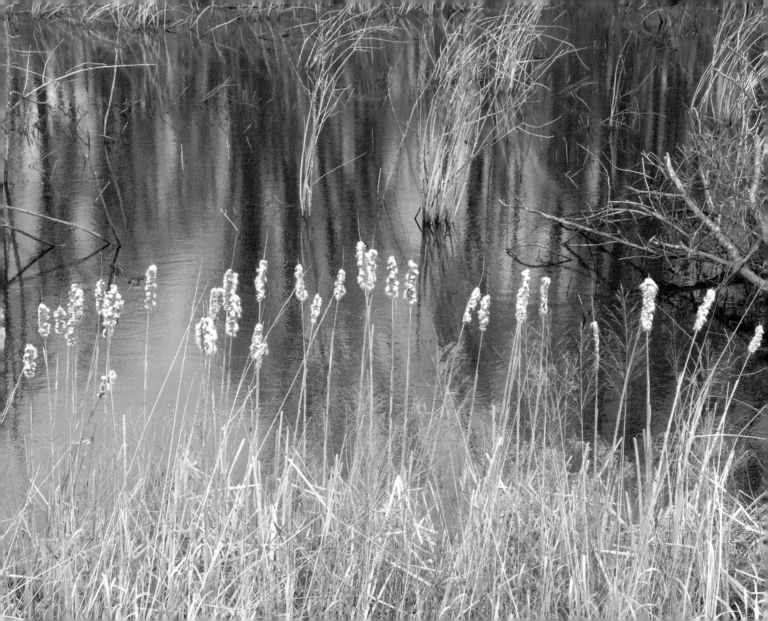

Oh Blessed Be

Love, efy

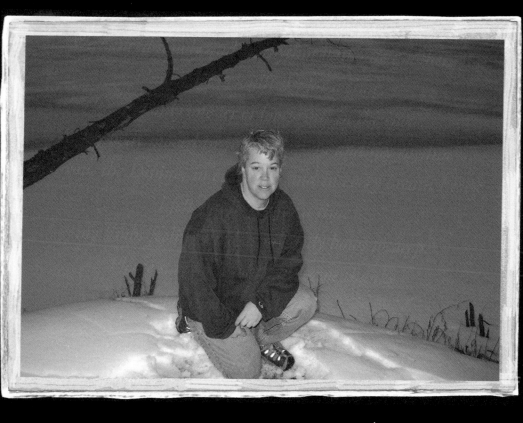

Photo of me by my son

With Gratitude

There are so many folks I want to thank. I'm thankful to my son and my former husband for their ongoing love and support for my path.

Thank you to my friends, Audra and Liz, who convinced me to go to HeartSong that first day when I was so sick to learn about Reiki.

To Jenny, who introduced me to Reiki, became my friend, and was there for me during my dying and rebirth. Jenny helped me heal. I'm thankful for the divine timing of this.

To Rich...and Mina for their beautiful friendship and love throughout this time.

To Dave and June, thank you for selling me your beautiful cabin at the lake and for being such wonderful neighbors and friends.

To Nancy and Jody who said my images were worthy – way back when I was so unsure. Thank you for your continued support on so many levels. And to the rest of my McDonald Niklaus family.

To my Mother who continued to love me and be supportive during the difficulties of healing. And to her husband Floyd for his loving kindness.

To my sister, Becky, who loved and supported me in so many ways...and to Connie. You are both blessings in my life.

To my community of friends in Cleveland and at Hope House of Prayer...who have been my family through so many changes. Thank you Tom and Carolyn and so many others, for your support.

To my previous family Christy, MaryJo, and Dan. Thank you for your support of me along the way. You will forever live in my heart.

To Sandy who, at a critical time during this process, reassured me of my sure-footedness and validated my path.

Mary, I'm so thankful for your friendship and for your family who always invites me in.

To Donna, a new friend, who lovingly read a draft of the book and in her supportive and caring way made important suggestions.

To Jan Phillips whose retreat at Kirkridge Retreat Center ["No Ordinary Time"- a multi-media, multi-sensory weekend] was AMAZING! I feel very blessed and thankful that I said Yes to going. There, I was presented with what I needed at just the right time. Thank you Jan, for leading such a beautiful time of sharing. Thank you to all who shared that sacred circle with me! You are all Blessing.

To the women I met at "Women's Voices for (a) Change" a three Day Body/Mind/Spirit Symposium for Women on using Creativity as a tool for Cultural Change, in Saratoga Springs, NY at Skidmore College. Jan Phillips invited me to share a slide show of my images with music during the symposium. Thank you to Jan and the LivingKindness Foundation for all the new connections who helped me bring this book to publication.

To Catherine for your creative inspiration and support and to Elsa for your creativity in designing my book.

And to Deborah who guided the editing process and made valuable suggestions. I'm thankful as she honored my voice throughout. Lovingly nudging and being ever so patient as we allowed the book to evolve in its own time and mine. And to our beautiful fruitful friendship that blossomed, during the many hours of our sharing. I am so happy that we are and have been on this path together. I love you Deb!